STEM CELLS - LABORATORY AND CLINICAL RESEARCH

Additional books in this series can be found on Nova's website
under the Series tab.

Additional E-books in this series can be found on Nova's website
under the E-books tab.

STEM CELLS - LABORATORY AND CLINICAL RESEARCH

INDUCED STEM CELLS

PATRICK J. SULLIVAN
AND
ELENA K. MORTENSEN
EDITORS

Nova Science Publishers, Inc.
New York

For permission to use material from this book please contact us:
Telephone 631-231-7269; Fax 631-231-8175
Web Site: http://www.novapublishers.com

Library of Congress Cataloging-in-Publication Data

Induced stem cells / editors, Patrick J. Sullivan and Elena K. Mortensen.
p. ; cm.
Includes bibliographical references and index.
ISBN 978-1-61324-613-9 (hardcover)
1. Stem cells. I. Sullivan, Patrick J. (Patrick Joseph), 1941- II. Mortensen, Elena K.
[DNLM: 1. Induced Pluripotent Stem Cells. QU 325]
QH588.S83I53 2011
616'.02774--dc23

2011015374

Published by Nova Science Publishers, Inc. † New York

Contents

Preface

Induced pluripotent stem (iPS) cell technology has paved new ways for disease modeling and drug discovery. Disease modeling with the differentiated neuronal cells from patient-specific iPS cells partially recapitulated the phenotypes of spinal muscular atrophy, familial dysautonomia and Rett syndrome. In this book, the authors present current research in the study of induced stem cells, including the cryopreservation of pluipotent stem cells; tissue engineering approaches using bioactive ceramics towards bone regeneration; induced pluripotent stem cell-derived hepatocytes as an alternative to human adult hepatocytes; iPS technology for studying neurodegenerative diseases and iPS from cord blood cells.

Chapter 1 - Regenerative medicine requires a large volume of target cells for cell transplantation in any individual procedure. The best way of fulfilling this requirement is to freeze the target cells (in this way they can be preserved for long periods), then to thaw them rapidly and supply them immediately. However, the cryopreservation of human pluripotent stem cells entails specific problems, such as the cellular fragility and cell death that occur with conventional cryopreservation methods; the lack of non-established method to obtain a large volume of cryopreserved cells, and the unknown effects of freezing on differentiated cells derived from pluripotent stem cells.

Since human embryonic stem (hES) cell lines were established in 1998, several freezing methods have been proposed and improved, and they have been applied to iPS cells, other stem cells as well as ES cells. From the historic viewpoint, the development of novel freezing methods can be divided into four categories: conventional methods using DMSO; vitrification using DMSO and other cryoprotectants; the introduction of the programmable freezer; and the use of the ROCK inhibitor, Y-27632 as a new cryoprotectant. The conventional method yielded poor results. Although the survival rate of thawed hES cells was less than 1%, it was considerably improved by the use of vitrification methods, especially with the newly introduced cryoprotectants. However, this required operators with advanced techniques that were able to perform the cryopreservation procedures rapidly, and it was not possible to cryopreserve a large volume of cells because of the restrictions imposed by the compromise between cooling volume and cooling velocity. A programmable freezer, in which a computer program controls the cooling rate so as to restrict supercooling, was introduced to improve the survival rate. Because this machine used liquid nitrogen, its operation was complicated and only a limited number of samples could be cryopreserved at the same time. Several problems of cryopreservation were solved by the introduction of Y-27632. When the hES cells were dissociated completely, most of them were dead. Therefore, hES cells were cryopreserved as colonies instead of single cells during the early development of cryopreservation methods, which lowered the survival rate. The introduction of Y-27632 enabled the convention of freezing only colonies of cells to be abandoned and proposed the novel method of cryopreservation of single hES or iPS cells such as mouse ES cells. This raised the expectations of more effective freezing methods, because the cryopreservation of cell clumps is more difficult than that of single cells. The necessary methodology has now been established and is becoming prevalent in stem cell research, and it will enable freezing of a large volume of human pluripotent cells. In this chapter, the authors trace the history of cryoprotocols associated with pluripotent stem cells and show how the trend is now again toward new slow cooling protocols that will replace the poorly performing slow cooling protocols that were used in the past.

Chapter 2 - Segmental bone defects resulting from trauma or pathological conditions represent formidable clinical challenges in orthopaedic surgery. Though current therapies include autografts and allografts or distraction osteogenesis, they are known for their inherent disadvantages like limited supply, increased morbidity, disease transmission potential and long term hospitalization respectively. In this context, tissue engineering becomes relevant for the treatment of large bone defects, where cells or growth factors are incorporated into a three-dimensional scaffold to mimic native tissue architecture and function in terms of osteoconduction, osteoinduction and osteointegration. Among the scaffolds, bioactive ceramics play an importance because of its similarity in chemical composition to bone. This review seeks to describe different tissue engineering approaches using bioactive ceramics towards bone regeneration in segmental bone defects. These include tissue-ingrowth (bioactive ceramics alone); cell transplantation (bioactive ceramics with mesenchymal stem cells) and signaling molecule (bioactive ceramics with growth factors).

Chapter 3 - Recent advances in induced pluripotent stem (iPS) cell research have attracted much attention. The ability to generate such cells from somatic cells has implications for overcoming both immunological rejection and the ethical issues associated with embryonic stem (ES) cells. Hepatocytes derived from patient-specific iPS cells offer a possible solution to the shortage of cell sources in cell replacement therapy, drug screening, and disease model. Despite such great promise, however, recent articles have questioned the viability of the therapeutic applications of iPS cells. These cells must, therefore, satisfy stringent criteria prior to practical use. The main focus of this review is a description of the current status of hepatic differentiation technology of iPS cells and a discussion of the concerns regarding the practical use of these techniques in cell replacement therapy, drug screening, and disease model. The current status of strategies for generating iPS cells and the accumulated knowledge on strategies for differentiating ES cells into hepatocytes will be summarized. The chapter also refers to the possibility of direct conversion of adult somatic cells into functional hepatocytes.

Chapter 4 – In 2006, it was reported that only four transcription factors were needed to remarkably reprogram mouse fibroblasts into cells similar to embryonic stem cells (ESCs) and those reprogrammed cells were named induced pluripotent stem cells (iPSCs). The year after, human iPSCs were produced and in 2008 reprogramming cells was chosen as the breakthrough of the year by Science magazine. In particular, this was due to the establishment of patient-specific cell lines from patients with various diseases using the induced pluripotent stem cell (iPSC) technique and also due to exciting scientific reports of direct reprogramming of somatic cells into other cell types, not necessary via a pluripotent cell state. The iPSCs can be generated by insertion of genes that turn back the developmental status of cells. These cells can be patient specific and therefore may prove useful in screens for potential drugs, regenerative medicine, increasing knowledge of human development, and in models for specific human diseases. This chapter provides a summary of cell types of human origin that have been transformed into iPSCs and of different iPSC procedures that exist. Further the authors discuss advantages and disadvantages of procedures, potential medical applications and implications that may arise in the iPSC field due to the resent report that reprogramming occurs using only retrovirus excluding transgenic transcription factors.

Chapter 5 - Induced pluripotent stem (iPS) cell technology has paved new ways for disease modeling and drug discovery. Disease modeling with the differentiated neuronal cells from patient-specific iPS cells partially recapitulated the phenotypes of spinal muscular atrophy (SMA), familial dysautonomia (FD) and Rett syndrome. Furthermore, proof of the efficacy of candidate drugs by iPS cell-based assay on SMA and FD has been reported.

There are several obstacles for disease modeling using iPS cell-derived neuronal cells. First, differentiated neuronal cells from patient-specific iPS cells might not be provoked sufficiently toward senescence to manifest the phenotype of late-onset diseases such as Parkinson disease (PD) and amyotrophic lateral sclerosis (ALS). Second, there are heterogeneous populations in cultured cells differentiated from iPS cells that might affect the disease phenotype. The propensity of various differentiations among iPS cells leads to the heterogeneity.

In this review, the authors will describe recent literature concerning the application of iPS cell technology for the study of neurological diseases and also discuss some experimental requirements.

Chapter 6 – This chapter reports that iPS cells can be safely and effectively generated from fresh human cord blood (CB) cells with Sendai virus (SeV) vector carrying reprogramming factors *OCT3/4, SOX2, KLF4,* and *c-MYC*. The SeV vector is a single strand RNA virus having no DNA phase, and selectively infects the freshly isolated $CD34^{+}$ $CD45^{low+}$ fraction of CB cells corresponding to hematopoietic progenitors. Approximately twenty ES cell-like colonies emerged from 1×10^{4} freshly isolated $CD34^{+}$ CB cells around 18 days after SeV infection and were selected for passage to reduce the frequency of the remaining SeV-infected cells. The complete elimination of viral constructs was confirmed after several passages by immunostaining with monoclonal antibody against hemagglutinin-neuraminidase (HN) and by RT-PCR analysis. Five ES cell-like clones were selected to examine their *in vitro* potential for three germ layer differentiation and their capacity for teratoma formation. Generation of non-integrating Sendai virus (SeV) iPS cells from CB cells may be an important step to provide allogeneic iPS cell-derived therapy in the future.

In: Induced Stem Cells
Editors: P. Sullivan and E. Mortensen
ISBN: 978-1-61324-613-9

Chapter I

Cryopreservation of Pluripotent Stem Cells: From Slow Cooling Protocols to Slow Cooling Protocols

Hinako Ichikawa and Katsunori Sasaki*
Department of Histology and Embryology, Organ Technology, Shinshu University School of Medicine

Abstract

Regenerative medicine requires a large volume of target cells for cell transplantation in any individual procedure. The best way of fulfilling this requirement is to freeze the target cells (in this way they can be preserved for long periods), then to thaw them rapidly and supply them immediately. However, the cryopreservation of human pluripotent stem cells entails specific problems, such as the cellular fragility and cell death that occur with conventional cryopreservation methods; the lack of non-established method to obtain a large volume of cryopreserved cells, and

* Corresponding Author:Katsunori Sasaki,M.D.,Ph.D.; Department of Histology and Embryology, Shinshu University School of Medicine, 3-1-1 Asahi, Matsumoto 390-8621, Japan, Phone: +81-263-37-2590, Fax: +81-263-37-3093, E-mail: katsmd@shinshu-u.ac.jp

the unknown effects of freezing on differentiated cells derived from pluripotent stem cells.

Since human embryonic stem (hES) cell lines were established in 1998, several freezing methods have been proposed and improved, and they have been applied to iPS cells, other stem cells as well as ES cells. From the historic viewpoint, the development of novel freezing methods can be divided into four categories: conventional methods using DMSO; vitrification using DMSO and other cryoprotectants; the introduction of the programmable freezer; and the use of the ROCK inhibitor, Y-27632 as a new cryoprotectant. The conventional method yielded poor results. Although the survival rate of thawed hES cells was less than 1%, it was considerably improved by the use of vitrification methods, especially with the newly introduced cryoprotectants. However, this required operators with advanced techniques that were able to perform the cryopreservation procedures rapidly, and it was not possible to cryopreserve a large volume of cells because of the restrictions imposed by the compromise between cooling volume and cooling velocity. A programmable freezer, in which a computer program controls the cooling rate so as to restrict supercooling, was introduced to improve the survival rate. Because this machine used liquid nitrogen, its operation was complicated and only a limited number of samples could be cryopreserved at the same time. Several problems of cryopreservation were solved by the introduction of Y-27632. When the hES cells were dissociated completely, most of them were dead. Therefore, hES cells were cryopreserved as colonies instead of single cells during the early development of cryopreservation methods, which lowered the survival rate. The introduction of Y-27632 enabled the convention of freezing only colonies of cells to be abandoned and proposed the novel method of cryopreservation of single hES or iPS cells such as mouse ES cells. This raised the expectations of more effective freezing methods, because the cryopreservation of cell clumps is more difficult than that of single cells. The necessary methodology has now been established and is becoming prevalent in stem cell research, and it will enable freezing of a large volume of human pluripotent cells. In this chapter, we trace the history of cryoprotocols associated with pluripotent stem cells and show how the trend is now again toward new slow cooling protocols that will replace the poorly performing slow cooling protocols that were used in the past.

Introduction

Human embryonic stem (hES) cell lines were established from fresh or frozen human blastocyst-stage embryos produced by in vitro fertilization for infertility therapy, after informed consent and IRB (institutional review board) approval in 1998 [1], and human induced pluripotent stem cells (hiPS cells) were generated from adult human dermal fibroblasts by the use of four factors–Oct3/4, Sox2, Klf4, and c-Myc in 2007 [2]. Since then, a large number of passaged cells have been frozen and preserved to maintain their undifferentiated state and pluripotency for long periods to satisfy the diverse requirements of basic research and regenerative medicine. Effective cryopreservation and thawing techniques are a fundamental requirement for all fields of study on living cells, but are not always easy to perform in hES research.

Freezing imposes a severe stress on all living cells and results in a considerable cell death owing to a combination of several factors. First, solution effects, i.e., when ice crystals are formed in freezing water, solutes are expelled from the ice crystals and concentrated in the water; this leads to cytodamage. Second, mechanical damage may occur because of extracellular ice formation. On slow cooling, intracellular water migrates into the extracellular space, where large amounts of ice are formed; this ice causes mechanical damage to the cellular membranes and intercellular junctions. Third, cellular dehydration due to migration of water may be followed by extracellular ice formation. Fourth, and most destructive, intracellular ice may be formed [3,4], unless ingenious countermeasures are taken. Once cells overcome these risks and reach the frozen stage, they may be preserved for approximately 1000 years; they could be revived without altering their intracellular material. However, the cells would have to be thawed, which is generally performed by rapid warming in a water bath set at 37°C, to revive them. Various cryopreservation techniques have been developed and improved for utilization in life sciences and reproductive medicine since 1949, when Polge et al. accidentally discovered that glycerol was an effective cryoprotectant [5]. However, the same method may not be applicable to all cells and a completely satisfactory method for individual cells has not yet been developed. In addition, suitable methods have not yet been developed for newly established or newly generated cells. Therefore, new cryopreservation techniques that are adapted to each cell type are needed. In this chapter, we trace the process of developing smart freezing methods since 1998. The chapter includes discussion of our new data and information on cryopreservation techniques suitable for hES cells and/or hiPS cells, and we offer a view into the future.

1. Poor Results of Conventional Slow Cooling Protocols

Solution effects, *extracellular* ice formation, cellular dehydration, and *intracellular* ice formation, which cause serious damage to living cells during cryopreservation—mainly during the freezing stage—can be minimized by using *cryoprotectants*. In the early years when hES cell lines were established, cells were frozen with conventional slow cooling protocols by using dimethyl sulfoxide (DMSO; $(CH_3)_2SO$), which was commonly used in the cryopreservation of mouse ES (mES) cells. DMSO, an excellent cryoprotectant, was first synthesized in 1866 and it was employed 80 years later in research life sciences. This compound rapidly penetrates cell membranes, replaces intracellular water, depresses the freezing point of intracellular water, reduces ice formation, and protects living cells from freezing damage and the deleterious effects of ice crystals [6]. Although the usage of DMSO was a routine, conventional method that was effective in mouse ES cells, with a post-thaw survival rate higher than 90% [7], the post-thaw survival rate of hES cells was extremely low. For example, the protocols of the WiCell Research Institute, as given in its introduction to human embryonic stem cell culture methods, states that recovery is approximately 0.1%–1% [cryopreservation medium consisted of 60% defined FBS, 20% hES cell culture medium and 20% DMSO]. Moreover, since the recovery rate after thawing is low, confirmation of visible colonies immediately after thawing may not be possible (WiCell and The WISC Bank - Home, www.wicell.org). In fact, the eight colonies we obtained after thawing an H1 cell line needed approximately 6 months to achieve problem-free passages and use the cells for researches [8]. To describe this method simply, clumps of ES cells consisting of about 100–200 cells were transferred into a 1.2 mL cryovial containing 0.5–1 mL precooled (4°C) freezing medium (90% serum and 10% DMSO). The vials were slowly cooled (approximately 1°C/minute) in a freezing container to –80°C and then plunged into and stored in liquid nitrogen. The vials were rapidly thawed in a water bath set at 37°C. The freezing medium was rapidly diluted with 7–8 mL ES cell culture medium. After centrifugation, thawed ES cell clumps were plated onto a fresh feeder layer. This was the beginning of all.

Several reports stated that conventional slow cooling protocols using standard concentrations of cryoprotectant (DMSO) yielded low survival rates: <5% [7,9,10], less than 1% [11], and 0% [12]. Heng et al. [13] confirmed by

TUNEL assay, immunocytochemical staining, and ultrastructural analysis that cell death in such conditions is due to apoptosis mediated through the enzymes of caspase family, and not cellular necrosis. As Kent [14] suggested, careful operations are required when freezing and thawing hES cells even in a conventional slow cooling protocol using 60% defined FBS, 20% hES cell culture medium, and 20% DMSO, before improving preexisting protocols.

Moreover, when slow cooling protocols are used hES cells deteriorate and yield fewer undifferentiated cells. Katkov et al. [15] froze an hES cell line containing an Oct-4 promoter-driven, enhanced green fluorescent protein (EGFP) reporter using 10% DMSO in a slow cooling protocol and preserved the cells in a freezer at −80°C for 3 days or 3 months. Although half of the cells frozen for 3 days were alive after thawing, only 10% demonstrated EGFP-/Oct-4 positivity. As time passed, the Oct-4-positive population increased, but large patches of EGFP-negative cells, i.e., a differentiated population remained within the clusters of colonies. This deleterious effect of freezing was more pronounced after 3 months of storage at −80°C. After 7 days of culture following thawing, only a few EGFP-positive cells observed. The authors suggested that slow cooling protocols using DMSO did not maintain complete undifferentiated state of cells, but whether this deterioration was due to the −80°C temperature or the slow cooling method with DMSO was not known. A different result may be obtained if the cells are preserved in liquid nitrogen.

The death of hES cells following the use of the slow cooling protocol, as suggested by Heng et al. [13], does not occur by necrosis but by apoptosis. However, such apoptosis does not begin directly after thawing. More than 90% of cells are alive immediately after thawing, and the number of dead cells increases with time. In our data, the peak of cell death occurs approximately 12 hours after thawing and cells continue to die for at least the subsequent 24 hours. It is important to find out why apoptosis in thawed hES cells begins gradually and continues for some time, and what facilitates this process. We will return to this topic later in this chapter.

2. And Yet We Continue to Use Slow Cooling Protocols

Continuous attempts have been made to improve conventional slow cooling protocolos even if they are unsuitable for hES cells because they are simple.

One strategy is to develop new cryoprotectants or to improve classic methods of reducing ice formation. The survival rate can be increased up to 10% with the optimal combination of 5%DMSO and 95%FBS [16]. Moreover, another optimal cryopreservation protocol for hES cells was developed using a combination of three cryoprotectants: DMSO, ethylene glycol (EG), and glycerol. When the percentages of DMSO, EG, and FBS were 5%, 10%, and 50%, respectively, the survival rate increased to approximately 30%. The key to the high level of efficiency of their protocol is the mixture of EG with DMSO and FBS. EG ($C_2H_6O_2$) was introduced by Miyamoto and Ishibashi [17] to freeze mouse and rat embryos by the conventional slow freezing method. EG shows rapid influx into living cells during equilibration and rapid efflux during dilution, and it functions effectively as a cryoprotectant. But few or no colonies were observed after adding 5% EG to 95% FBS; 10% EG to 90% FBS; 5% EG to 5% DMSO–50% FBS; or 20% EG to 5% DMSO–50% FBS. This suggests that a fixed concentration of EG is required in addition to its combination with other cryoprotectants to reduce ice formation. After hES cells cryopreserved by this technique were thawed, the surviving cells maintained the inherent characteristics of human ES cells, including the undifferentiated state and pluripotency.

The disaccharide trehalose ($C_{12}H_{22}O_{11}$;alpha-D-glucopyranoside and alpha-D-glucopyranosyl) is well known as an excellent cryoprotectant that can stabilize the cellular membrane, reduce ice formation, and replace water [18]. Wu et al. [19] added 0.2 mol/L of trehalose to a freezing medium containing 90% knockout serum replacement (KSR) and 10% DMSO at the thawing stage or in both the freezing and the thawing medium and obtained excellent recovery rates, 42% or 48%, respectively compared to that of the freezing medium (37%), though good preservation of hES cells seemed to be achieved in the freezing medium as well. The thawed cells retained pluripotency with a normal karyotype.

Another interesting strategy is to combine the extracellular matrix (ECM) or its components with cryoprotectants on the basis that the ECM influences various cellular functions, including growth, differentiation, and apoptosis, in hES cells [20]. When type IV collagen (1 μg/mL) was added to the freezing medium (90% KSR, 10% DMSO), the survival rate of hES cells after thawing increased to 36% compared with 22% in the control (freezing medium without collagen). Furthermore, in contrast to the survival rate, the differentiate rate (assessed on the basis of morphological appearance: undifferentiated areas consisted of small cells with a high nucleus-to-cytoplasm ratio; differentiated areas consisted of large cells with abundant cytoplasm) decreased to one-third of the rate in the frozen control (35%); however, additional evidence other than morphological data will be required to confirm this effect.

Ji et al. [21] developed a unique technique. They cultured hES cell lines in a 24-well plate in a growth medium containing 0.25 mg of Matrigel matrix in each well for 2 days; they replaced the medium with the freezing medium [10% DMSO, 30% FBS, and 60% MEF-conditioned medium including bFGF]; then they immediately froze the plate at −80°C at a cooling rate of −1°C/minute. The number of viable cells adhering to the plate was 14 times that of cells in suspension in the freezing medium. They put such an efficiency on the base that hES colonies get ECM signaling continuously after thawing, because they continue to attach the plate . In addition to the use of Matrigel matrix, loading adherent hES cells with 35 mM of disaccharide trehalose 24 h before cryopreserving them in a cryoprotectant solution containing 10% DMSO-50–90% FBS further increases cell viability by 25% compared with cryopreserving them solely in DMSO. However, as Heng et al. [7] suggested, long-term storage is not possible using this technique because it is difficult to preserve the plate in liquid nitrogen; therefore, they proposed to redesign the incorporated culture plate with detachable wells with screw caps that are resistant to low temperatures. In addition, Heng et al. [7] do not clarify why suspended colonies do not adhere to the plate after thawing. This interesting issue will be discussed later in this chapter.

3. Why are Human ES Cells Vulnerable to Conventional Slow Cooling Protocols?

The above techniques are good for neither one thing nor the other. An important clue that may enable us to solve this problem is that although slow cooling protocols are effective in mES cells, they are ineffective in hES cells. If the various issues related to conventional slow cooling techniques are brought into relief, opportunities to invent new countermeasures may present themselves.

A. How do mES Cells and hES Cells Differ?

hES cells have unique features that are different from those of mES cells. Cellular dissociation is fatal to hES cells, which are able to survive only as a colony, as seen in the early work on the establishment of hES lines [22,23]. This is because hES cells need intimate physical contact and paracrine signaling among themselves [7,13]. The mechanisms that maintain the characteristic cooperation observed in hES cells and how these mechanisms are disrupted during freezing procedures, culminating in cell death, have not yet been confirmed. However, according to Amit et al. [22] the presence of serum components is detrimental to stem cell survival when the colonies are dispersed to single cells.

B. What Happens in Cellular Clumps During Conventional Slow Cooling Protocols?

Heng et al. [7] summarized the damaging events or mechanisms seen in ES colonies after thawing as follows. In the case of cell clumps, the freezing medium may not penetrate uniformly into the interior of the clump, which in turn may reduce the post-thaw viability of living cells that do not receive adequate exposure to the medium. The relatively extensive ice crystallization in conventional slow cooling protocols inflicts severe cellular damage, resulting in dissociation of the intercellular junctions formed among hES cells, which play an important role in maintaining cooperative interactions through tight and gap junctions [24] and considerable changes in the osmolarity and pH of the aqueous solution due to ice formation. These pernicious events are further exacerbated by prolonged exposure of hES cells to the cryopreservation solution in conventional slow cooling protocols, probably because of the toxicity of the cryoprotectants.

Unfortunately, we do not know what happens in the cryovial containing hES colonies during conventional slow cooling, especially in the thermoregulated environment in which living cells become frozen; we need to be mindful of all events to devise new, effective countermeasures. To investigate the cooling curve in the freezing medium, a thermosensor was directly inserted into a cryovial filled with a medium consisting of 10% (v/v) DMSO, 20% (v/v) FBS, and 70% IMDM, which was transferred into a precooled Bicell freezing vessel kept at −80°C. Figure 1 shows three types of cooling curve.

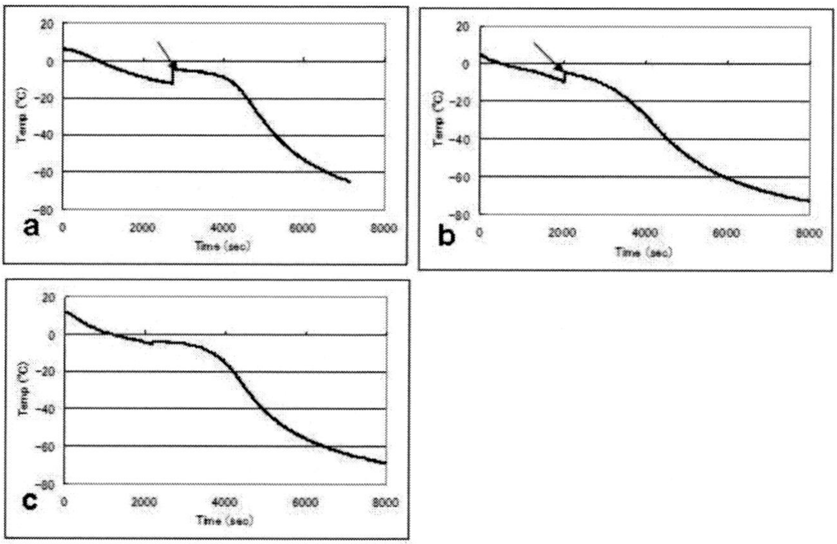

Figure 1. Three types of cooling temperature curves in a. conventional slow cooling protocol in the same condition. a. Marked supercooling. b. Small supercooling. c. No supercooling .

The first curve in Fig. 1 shows an acute increase to −3.5°C after the temperature drops to −11°C at 45 minutes after the start of cooling. In the second curve there is a similar phenomenon, occurring at 33 minutes, but the extent of the increase in temperature is small: 4.3°C. This increase is barely detectable in the third curve. The small rise—less than 1°C—occurs at 33 minutes. This abrupt rise in temperature seen in frozen events is due to the well-known phenomenon of supercooling, in which a liquid freezes abruptly and spontaneously at a temperature below the standard freezing point. An abrupt, rapid increase in temperature is caused by the release of latent heat followed by ice formation from the liquid [25]. Consequently, the stability of the cytoplasm and intercellular junctions in the supercooling condition is suddenly disrupted. Ice crystals form and increase in size, and this damages the intracellular structures and intercellular junctions. However, the three cooling curves show that the temperature rise is lesser when supercooling time is shorter or when the extent of the temperature decrease is smaller. In addition, the unregulated supercooling that occurs in conventional slow cooling protocols may be fatal to living cells in cell clumps, but it does not always lower the survival rate of single cells, as seen in mES cells. Both these facts must be taken into consideration when devising new cryopreservation protocols.

C. Main Intercellular Junctions of hES Cells: E-Cadherins

When hES cell colonies are enzymatically or mechanically dissociated into single cells, most single cells lose their proliferative ability, do not colonize, and die sooner or later. To provide conditions in which single hES cells can proliferate and retain an undifferentiated state is an important requirement for successful cryopreservation, because cryoprotectants penetrate all cells equally and help freeze them more effectively, as seen in mES cells. To supply functional single hES cells for the development of cryopreservation techniques, we need to know what happens in dissociated hES cells. Dissociation is followed directly by disruption of the intercellular junctions. First, knowledge of the junctions formed between hES cells is important. In an ultrastructural study, Santhananthan et al. [24] found desmosomes anchored by tonofilaments. Gap junctions were well developed among hES cells and played important roles in the survival and differentiation of hES cells. Expression of the genes for connexins (Cx) 25, 26, 30.3, 31, 31.1, 31.9, 37, 40, 43, 45, and 46 was detected by reverse transcription–polymerase chain reaction [26]. Immunohistochemical examination confirmed that the proteins Cx40, 43, and 45 were dotted around the cellular periphery and this distribution was supported by a fine structure study [26,27]. Use of the dye injection method showed that direct intercellular communication among hES cells was established through these gap junctions; however, communication was disrupted between hES and feeder cells [26]. Gap junctions among hES cells mediated the transport of shRNA [28] and were inhibited by protein kinase C activation and extracellular signal-regulated kinase inhibition [29]. When the decoupling agent alpha-glycyrrhetinic acid was used to close gap junctions in a hES cell monolayer, hES colonies ceased growing and showed an increase in cell apoptosis [30,31]. These data indicate that gap junctions may play an important role in the cooperative nature of hES cells; the loss of gap junctions, followed by cellular dissociation, may result in apoptosis. Gap junctions themselves are soon reformed and a clump of cells begins to form if a single cell adheres to another. Re-adhesion after dissociation is a necessary factor for the establishment of cooperative behavior among hES cells. Furthermore, the gap junction is not a suitable candidate for facilitating re-adhesion, because these junctions are not formed over the entire cell surface but are dotted around the periphery of the cell [26,29].Of the cell–cell adhesion molecules identified by a mass spectrometry-based plasma membrane proteome analysis of hES cells cultured as monolayers, E-cadherins (zonula adherens); junctional adhesion molecule A (tight junction); desmoglein-2 preproprotein, desmoplakin isoform (desmosome); and Cx43 (gap junction) showed high Mascot scores [32]. In addition to the abovementioned desmosomes, tight junctions, and gap junctions, the hES cells formed zona adherence through E-cadherins, anchored by actin filaments. Here we will focus on E-cadherins because the role of tight junctions in cell death associated with cellular dissociation is not well documented. These adhesion molecules are closely associated with embryonic stages, expressed dominantly in the undifferentiated stage, and replaced by N-cadherins when the developmental process progresses from the undifferentiated to the differentiated stage [33]. Use of the immunofluorescence-assisted affinity mapping (IF-AM) method has shown that the expression of E-cadherins is considerably higher in undifferentiated cells (the number of E-cadherins/μm^2 is approximately 200 in the undifferentiated state, 90 in the endoderm, 40 in the mesoderm, and 10 in the ectoderm) and that the distribution of E-cadherins in hES cells is relatively homogeneous [34]. Overall expression of E-cadherins in hES cells suggests that these adhesion molecules play an important role in the formation of intercellular junctions and colonies of cells. Another line of research has shown that greater abundance of E cadherins is associated with a high likelihood of cell agglomeration and subsequent survival in suspension [35]. Li et al. [36] investigated factors affecting the clonogenicity of hES cells and offered two interesting observations about the role of E-cadherins in colony formation. Inhibition of Rho-associated kinase considerably upregulated hES cell reaggregation, producing considerable number of false-positive colonies; however, E-cadherin upregulation considerably augmented hES cell clonogenicity through improved survival of single ES cells. Rap1 is necessary in the endocytic recycling pathway, which is involved in the formation and maintenance of E-cadherin-mediated cell–cell cohesion and the normal functions of E-cadherins—colony formation and self-renewal [36]. These data suggest that E-cadherins are intimately related to re-adhesion and cell survival after dissociation, and they are intricately regulated by Rho kinase [37].

Moreover, E-cadherins, which are intramembrane proteins, are regulated through anchor proteins by cytoplasmic actin filaments. Therefore, it is speculated that pathological conditions of cytoplasmic actin filaments interrupt cell–cell adhesion and colony formation of hES cells, leading to cell death. This idea is supported by recent reports. Chen et al. [38] reported that actin–myosin contraction had a critical effect on the cell death response to the dissociation of hES cells. Inhibition of myosin heavy chain ATPase and downregulation of myosin light and heavy chains increased cell survival and cloning efficiency. ROCK inhibitors decrease phosphorylation of the myosin light chain, which results in inhibition of actin–myosin contraction and increases the cloning efficacy of hES cells. Ohgushi et al. [39] showed that the Abr-dependent Rho-high/Rac-low state played a decisive role in dissociation-induced actomyosin hyperactivation and apoptosis in hES cells. Non-muscle myosin II (NMMII) is necessary for E-cadherin-mediated intercellular adhesion, mechanical tension, and p120-catenin function [40]. Treatment with an inhibitor of NMMII such as blebbistatin enhances the survival and self-renewal of human pluripotent stem cells under single-cell conditions [41]. These reports show that E-cadherins are closely associated with apoptosis through actomyosin hyperactivation after dissociation, but give no indication about why hES cells are vulnerable to freezing, how apoptotic events progress, and how E-cadherins are distributed during the freezing and thawing of hES cells. In particular, the reason why apoptosis occurs in association with cryopreservation as well as with dissociation, and the nature of the trigger of apoptosis remain elusive.

What happens in hES cell clumps during freezing–thawing processes in conventional cooling protocols is very simple. After thawing of hES cells frozen using this method, no intact fine cell clumps are found. Single ES cells or clumps consisting of only a few cells predominate. Intercellular separation due to extracellular ice formation in conventional slow cooling protocols occurs in hES cell clumps during freezing–thawing. Another possible explanation of this phenomenon is that it takes more time for hES cells to adhere to the plate after thawing, unlike the time taken after passaging. Immediately after thawing, hES cells do not readily adhere to plates prepared using MEF, which suggests that freezing–thawing has a marked effect on cellular adhesion.

On the basis that maintenance of E-cadherins after dissociation facilitates prompt re-adhesion of hES cells and suppresses the apoptotic events that occur in individual hES cells and the intercellular separation that commonly occurs in hES cell cryopreservation, some strategies for improving cryopreservation techniques were proposed. One strategy is to suppress intercellular separation; another is to rescue separated cells that are dying. A unique method was proposed by Ji et al. [21]. When an ES colony was frozen without separating it from the plate, E-cadherins were completely preserved; however, this method is not practical for many laboratories. To prevent extracellular ice formation, it is necessary to minimize ice crystallization in addition to ensuring equal penetration of cryoprotectants into all living cells. Another idea is to cryopreserve a single hES cell with intact E-cadherin function and suppression of actomyosin hyperactivation. This method seems feasible and is discussed later in this chapter.

Before ending this section, we will consider anoikis that is another cause of cell death in addition to dissociation and freezing. Anoikis is a form of apoptosis and is induced by the loss of cell adhesion or by inappropriate cell adhesion and often occurs on detachment of cells from the ECM [4]. However, if the colony becomes detached from the substrate, it is not fatal to hES cells. Ohgushi et al. [39] reported that the apoptosis that occurred in hES cells after disassociation was of the non-anoikis type. hES cell colonies were removed by scraping and stained with Trypan Blue; Fig. 2 shows that the periphery of the colony was stained, but most cells in the colony were alive and unstained. These colonies formed embryoid bodies in non-adherent plates and did not show cell death.

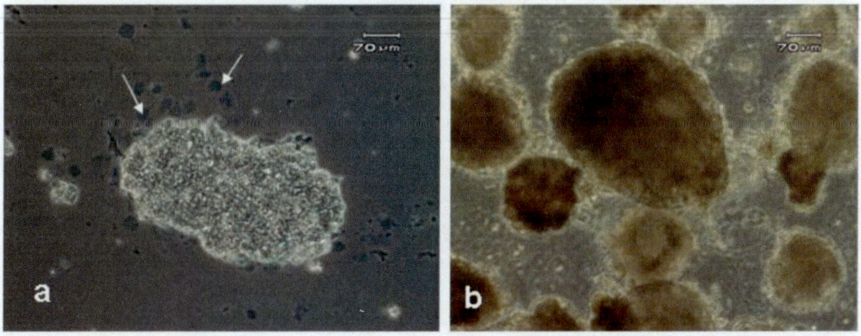

Figure 2. After the colony becomes separated from the plate by the scraper mechanically, it is stained with trypan blue. Most cells forming the colony are still alive, but individual cells (arrows) are dead. b. After floating in the non-adherent plate for some time, it forms an embryoid body.

3. Does the Survival Rate of hES Cells After Thawing Increase if Supercooling is Regulated?

A liquid below its freezing point crystallizes in the presence of a seed crystal or nucleus. If it does not contain any seed nuclei, however, the liquid phase is maintained until the temperature at which crystal homogeneous nucleation occurs that is attained by quick cooling. For pure water this temperature is approximately −42°C. One strategy to avoid abnormal ice formation and prevent cytodamage is to regulate supercooling, acquire crystal homogeneous nucleation, and minimize crystal size. This method is called controlled-rate slow freezing or slow programmable freezing. It was established in the early 1970s and was in general use in the field of reproductive medicine for a long period. The principal requirements of this method are the controlled cooling rate and the controlled seeding point; the only device that can satisfy these requirements is a programmable freezer. A study in which pancreatic islets as well as blastocysts were frozen with a programmable freezer and showed a high survival rate encouraged us to freeze hES colonies with such a device [43], because similar to the hES, the islets and blastocysts formed cell clumps.

It is generally said that a typical cooling rate of approximately 1°C/minute is appropriate for many living cells after treatment with cryoprotectants, but this is not a universal optimum rate. Samples were frozen in the freezing containers within the range of 0.35–1.57°C/minute without using a programmable freezer, but it was followed by an abrupt temperature increase of 10°C(supercooling). Conditions such as cooling speed and seeding point have been determined according to the cell type to achieve crystal homogenous nucleation, although the conditions have not been individually determined in each laboratory.

Figure 3 shows an example where samples were cooled at 2°C/minute to −5°C and were maintained at that temperature for 20 minutes to set the seeding point to −40°C. Then, they were cooled at 0.3°C/minute to −30°C, whereupon the cooling rate was increased to 50°C/minute down to −100°C. The cooling curve shows an absence of the abrupt temperature increase that is seen in conventional slow cooling (Fig. 1).

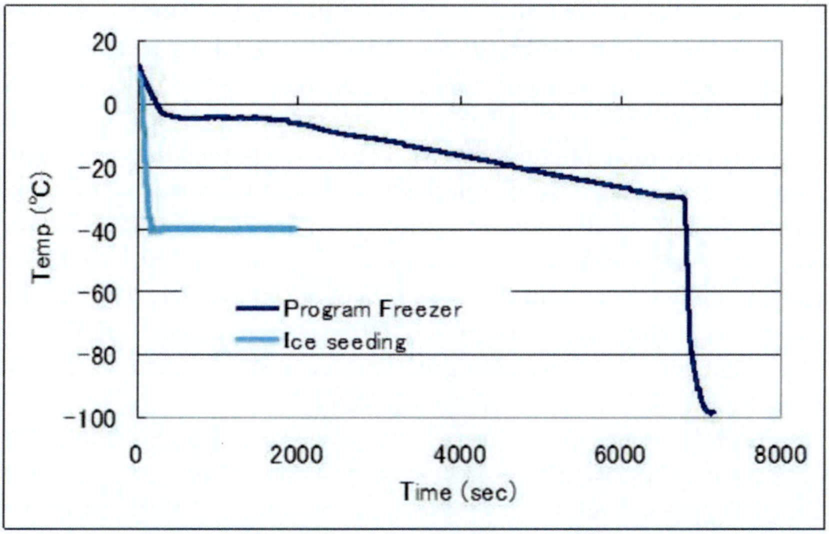

Figure 3. Cooling curve in a programable freezer. Surpercooling does not occur if ice seeding is induced.

Although cytodamage because of ice crystallization is minimized by reducing the size of ice crystals through a controlled rate of slow cooling and setting the seeding point, Heng et al. [7] referred to the study by Richards et al. [44] in their review and suggested that slow cooling with a programmable freezing device is not as effective as might be expected, because the procedure may extend the duration of exposure of the cells to the cytotoxic effects of cryoprotectants. However, the method of crystal homogeneous nucleation has important merits. If discouraging results are obtained with this method, it may be because the necessary conditions, which are complicated, have not been determined correctly or because the best use is not being made of the device. Yang et al. [45,46] reported that a high survival rate (approximately 82%) was obtained when a sample was suspended in the freezing medium containing 10%DMSO, 30%FBS, and 60%DMEM was cooled from 0°C to −35°C at the rate of 0.5°C/minute with a seeding temperature of −10°C. Moreover, Ware et al. [47] obtained survival rates of 20%–80% and reported that the critical factors for the highest survival rate were an ice crystal seed (at −7° to −10°C) and a freezing rate between 0.3–1.8°C/minute. Ware et al. developed another programmed freezing method using straws. An ice crystal seed was induced at −10°C, and this was followed by controlled cooling at −1°C/minute down to −33°C, with a direct plunge into liquid nitrogen that was at −196°C. Rapid thawing was effected by moving the frozen cells directly from liquid nitrogen into a water bath and transferring them directly into culture medium without stepwise cryoprotectant removal. Using this improved protocol, the survival of hES cells increased from 1% or less to approximately 80% [48]. Lee et al. [49] developed a new method combining stepwise equilibration using a program-controlled freezer: stepwise equilibration comprised immersion of samples initially in the ES medium containing 50% serum replacement (SR), secondly in 90% SR and 5% DMSO, and finally in 90%) SR and 10% DMSO; the samples were then transferred to the programmable freezer and frozen to −80°C with a seeding temperature of −7°C and a cooling rate of −1°C/minute, and then plunged into liquid nitrogen. The survival rate increased to 30%–50%. However, this protocol is very complicated.

To reconfirm the superiority of this device for freezing multicellular clumps, we froze mouse embryoid bodies consisting of three germ cell layers following the same conditions as those shown in Fig. 3 [50]. The survival rate of embryoid bodies was twice that obtained with the usual slow cooling protocol, and pluripotency was maintained. hES cells were frozen by the same protocol. The survival rate was approximately 60% and twice that of the control. Colonies obtained after thawing were compacted and adhered to the plate within 24 hours. They proliferated rapidly and showed no difference in morphology after repeated passages. As mentioned above, several reports have confirmed that slow programmable freezing with artificial seeding and a conventional cryoprotectant is effective in freezing cell clumps.

The method has several drawbacks, however, including the difficulty of operating the device, the necessity for liquid nitrogen for cooling, which causes problems with the device, and excessive time required for the completion of freezing. Only few cryovials can be handled at the same time. As bulk freezing is difficult with this method, it may not be practical for regenerative medicine, which requires a large volume of living cells. The invention of a powerful electrical refrigerator that can rapidly cool not only cryovials but large bags and does not require liquid nitrogen will be a breakthrough in regenerative medicine. Bulk freezing is the final goal in pluripotent stem cell cryopreservation.

Recently, Li et al. [51] reported that programmable cryopreservation and vitrification methods are appropriate for the cryopreservation of hES cells, whereas the conventional slow freezing method is not appropriate, although vitrification resulted in higher attachment and recovery rates compared with the other two methods.

4. What is Vitrification?

In some regulated conditions, the supercooling of pure water stops at −42°C and shifts to homogeneous nucleation devoid of impurities [52]. Between −123°C and −137°C crystallization to cubic ice occurs. The final stage is glassy water, i.e., vitrification. The transition occurs at −108°C if crystallization to cubic ice is avoided. Vitrification is not followed by ice formation and avoids intracellular and extracellular cytodamage due to ice crystals. To achieve vitrification, however, stringent conditions must be satisfied. Samples must be uniformly cooled below −108°C at the same time and a cooling velocity greater than 20,000°C/minute is necessary [53].

Water vitrifies without ice crystal formation. Using yeast, Moor and *Mühlethaler [54]* showed that cooling rate was closely associated with the survival rate of the cells. The survival rate was 1% at −10°C/second (quick freezing), 30% at −100°C/minute (snap freezing), and approximately 100% at −10000°C/minute (liquid helium). In all cases in which the survival rate exceeded 50%, the pores produced by ice crystals in the cytoplasm were absent or too small (10 nm or less) to be detected.

Interestingly, vitrification has been introduced in the field of morphology as an excellent fixation technique, because this technique preserves the ultrastructure and intracellular materials much better than chemical fixation. However, continuous attempts have been made to overcome a serious limitation of vitrification. Understanding of this limitation will in turn lead to understanding of the requirements of cryopreservation of living cells by vitrification. Various cryotechniques, such as immersion freezing, high-pressure freezing, spray freezing, jet freezing, plunge freezing, and copper block freezing, have been developed to preserve fine ultrastructure without chemical fixation [55,56]. Among these methods, copper block freezing (the metal contact or metal mirror method) is a reliable method; this method yields excellent physical fixation by rapidly impacting a sample to the polished surface of precooled metal block with high thermal conductivity, preserving proteins in addition to ultrastructure [57,58,59,60], but the glass-like state is restricted to a thin zone at the surface of the specimen. The depth of vitrification of the living cells and tissues is extremely small—between approximately 10 μm when liquid nitrogen is used and 30 μm when liquid helium is used [57,61]. With ultra-rapid cooling, vitrification is complete even in water, but the depth of vitrification is extremely shallow. Only three layers of cells can be vitrified by this method.Therefore, it is not practical in routine cryopreservation.

A relatively large surface-to-volume ratio is required for uniform cooling and cryoprotectant penetration. The first strategy is to increase the surface area and reduce the volume. This is why the straw method has been developed. This method will be discussed later in this chapter.

Another strategy is to replace intracellular water with liquids such as cryoprotectants that assume a glass-like state without ice formation, because vitrification occurs when the viscosity of the solution reaches a value at which it inhibits the crystallization of ice [62]. For example, Elford and Walter [63] performed a stepwise increase in the concentration of DMSO to 60% during slow cooling of smooth muscle to −79°C in unfrozen Krebs-based DMSO solution and avoided ice crystal formation with prompt recovery in potassium-rich media after rewarming. DMSO is the most fundamental, effective protectant in vitrification. Many cryoprotectants have been developed based on DMSO.

A. Is Vitrification Effective in hES Cell Clump Freezing?

Reubinoff et al. [64] first introduced vitrification methods in ES cell biology using the open straw method. Apart from the present study, Richards et al. [44] and Zhou et al. [65] compared vitrification with the conventional slow cooling protocol and indicated the superiority of vitrification, giving survival rates higher than 75%.The freezing containers generally used in vitrification are special open or closed cryostraws. Vajta et al. [53] developed this novel technique and applied it to the cryopreservation of bovine ova and embryos. Ministraws (250 µl) are heat-softened over a hotplate and pulled manually until the inner diameter and the wall thickness are about one-half of the original values. Ova or embryos are loaded into the narrow end of the straw from a droplet by means of the capillary effect. Cooling is performed by direct plunging into liquid nitrogen. At thawing, the straws are immersed directly into the medium; the vitrification medium then liquifies and is immediately diluted by the holding medium, which enters the straw because of capillarity. Subsequently, the ova or embryos emerge from the straw into the culture plate through sedimentation.

Reubinoff et al. [64] modified this protocol slightly, as follows: four to six clumps of ES cells are first incubated in vitrification solution including 10%

DMSO and 10% EG for 1 minute, followed by incubation in the next vitrification solution, which contains 20% DMSO, 20% EG, and 0.5 mol/L sucrose, for 25 seconds. The clumps are loaded into the narrow end of the straw from the droplet by capillarity. The narrow end is immediately plunged into liquid nitrogen and preserved. In thawing, 3 seconds after removal from liquid nitrogen the narrow end of the straw is submerged into the holding medium containing 0.2 mol/L sucrose. The wide opening of the straw is sealed when a drop of the medium at the tip of the straw has liquefied and the straw begins to get filled with medium. Expansion of cold air in the straw because of the gradual increase in temperature leads to expulsion of the cell clumps into the plate. After 1 minute of incubation, the clumps are transferred and further incubated for 5 minutes in the holding medium containing 0.1 mol/L sucrose. The clumps are further incubated twice in the holding medium before being plated onto a fresh feeder layer. All hES cell clumps that were vitrified by the open pulled straw method could be recovered upon thawing, and gave rise to ES cell colonies after plating. Vitrified colonies were significantly smaller and showed an increased level of background differentiation compared with control colonies. However, these unwanted effects could be overcome by additional cultivation of colonies for 1 and 2 days, respectively. The vitrified hES cells were cultivated for prolonged periods and they retained pluripotency. 70% of the clumps could be recovered after thawing, and only 16% developed after plating into undersized ES cell colonies with a high level of differentiation. Prolonged culture (2 weeks) was required to allow proliferation of undifferentiated cells in the minority of these colonies.

The protocol developed by Zhou et al. [65] is almost similar to that by Reubinoff et al. [64] with slight modifications in the concentration of sucrose in the vitrification and thawing solutions, which decreases the extracellular osmotic pressure, affecting the vitrified ES cells and the number of ES clumps (10–15) vitrified at one time. In their study, the survival rate of vitrified ES cell clumps was 82%. All the recovered clumps produced colonies after plating; 34% of the colonies remained predominantly undifferentiated. In the slow freezing group, 16 of 70 ES cell clumps (23%) were recovered, and only one undifferentiated colony (6%) was obtained after plating. These data indicate that vitrified ES cells have greater potential for proliferation and remaining undifferentiated than cells frozen slowly. According to Reubinoff et al. [64] and Zhou et al. [65], significant levels of spontaneous differentiation were observed after thawing, because of cell injury, cryoprotectants, or dissociation of small cell clumps (<20 cells). Usually, however, hES colonies revert to a completely undifferentiated state with advanced culture techniques after a few passages.

One disadvantage of the open pulled straw method was indicated by Richards et al. [44]. It is non-sterile because the cell-containing medium contacts the liquid nitrogen directly and is exposed to the potential hazard of transmission of infective agents, such as contamination with hepatitis B virus because of the leakage of the cryopreservation bags in the liquid nitrogen tank [66], although no evidence of any contamination was observed during prolonged cultivation after vitrification [64]. Unexpected infectious contamination may be caused by direct contact not only with liquid nitrogen but also with xenoserum e.g., FBS. Richards et al. [44] proposed three countermeasures to avoid contamination and develop an effective, safe, and sterile cryopreservation protocol: sealed closed straws (CSs); storage of straws in the vapor phase of liquid nitrogen; and the replacement of FBS with human serum albumin. According to their protocol, five to eight dissected colony fragments of hES cells consisting of approximately 300–400 cells in vitrification solution containing 20% DMSO and 20% EG were loaded into the straw with one end sealed with a cotton plug after complicated manipulation. Holding the straw with a pair of precooled forceps, both ends of the straw were sealed with a plastic bag heat sealer. Then, it was plunged into and stored in either the liquid or vapor phase of liquid nitrogen. To thaw vitrified straws, the straws were removed from storage and then plunged immediately into a beaker containing water at room temperature. After the columns in the straw were thawed (approximately 5 seconds) and swabbed with a 70% isopropanol sterile wipe, the sealed ends of the straw were cut off with sterile scissors. The entire content of the straw was expelled into the washing solution. With this method survival rate was approximately 75%–88%, compared with 8% after conventional slow freezing. Vitrified-warmed colonies were observed to differentiate slightly earlier than unfrozen control colonies; they exhibited low differentiation rates, remained pluripotent, and maintained normal diploid karyotypes throughout an extended passage.

These methods using very small carriers are restricted to large volumes of cells. Fujioka et al. [67] overcame this problem by changing the components of the cryoprotectant in vitrification solution to include 2 M DMSO, 1 M acetamide, and 3 M propylene glycol without stepwise processing and with conventional cryovials. To thaw the vitrified ES cells, the medium was prewarmed to 37°C and added to the vials. The cells were thawed quickly by pipetting after centrifugation. Vitrification and thawing were performed within 30 seconds because of the toxicity of the cryoprotectant. Using standard slow cooling methods, the cryopreservation efficiency for monkey ES cell lines was approximately 0.4%, whereas that for a human ES cell line was almost 0%. Primate ES cell lines, however, were successfully cryopreserved by this vitrification method using conventional cryovials; this yielded a survival rate of approximately 6.5% for monkey ES cells and 12.2% for hES cells. Vitrified ES cells quickly recovered after thawing and exhibited the same morphology as non-vitrified cells. In addition, they retained a normal karyotype and continued to express ES cell markers after thawing. In our laboratory, ES cells are mainly cryopreserved according to these protocols (Fig. 4).

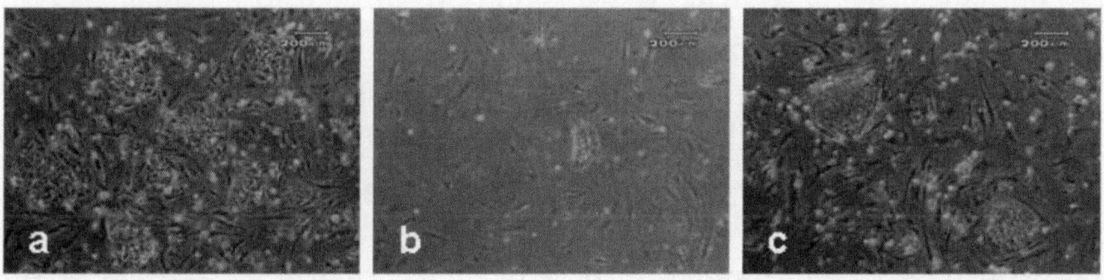

Figure 4. Colony formation after vitrification. The rate of colony formation differs among cell line. a. It ishigher in KhES 1. b. It is lower in KhES 2. c. KhES3 is the same as KhES1.

Although the survival rate of this method is lower than with other vitrification methods and programmable freezer protocols, the protocols are simple, not too laborious and adequate for routine research purposes. In our experience, however, rapid manipulation within 30 seconds, particularly in thawing, is relatively difficult to accomplish. In addition, the cellular response to cryopreservation techniques differ among cell lines, as seen in Fig. 4.

B. What are the Disadvantages of Vitrification?

Vitrification techniques minimize the exposure time of the cells to low temperatures outside the normal physiological temperature range, circumvent problems associated with ice formation and cell dehydration, and eliminate the formation of ice crystals; they are extremely laborious and it is difficult to handle bulk quantities of cells using this technique [68]. Carriers such as those used for vitrification, such as electron microscope grids [69], straws [44,64,65], and cryoloops, consisting of a nylon loop (20 µm wide; 0.5–0.7 mm diameter) [70,71], are very small. Cryopreservation of large volumes of cells is difficult, which seriously hinders the establishment and development of regenerative medicine. This is mainly because these tiny carriers cannot even hold surplus hES cell colonies during routine passage, let alone the large numbers of hES cells that might be propagated and cryopreserved in a scheduled study. Moreover, transferring cell clumps from one plate to another using Pasteur pipettes is time-consuming and might cause toxic and osmotic damage to cells. The development of regenerative medicine may be fatally hampered if vitrification cannot deal with bulk volumes.

To overcome these limitations, Li et al. [72] attempted bulk vitrification. They introduced a cell strainer (70 μm nylon) for this purpose, which was cup-shaped and made of nylon mesh. Small clumps (diameter <70 μm) were washed through this cell strainer and therefore excluded from cryopreservation. Each cell strainer was loaded with colonies harvested from half of a 35 mm plate (approximately 136 cell clumps), which was 30 times more than the colonies loaded in a pulled straw in open pulled straw group (approximately 4 cell clumps), instead of straws and other carriers; a final vitrification solution containing 20% DMSO, 20% EG, and 0.5 mol/L sucrose was added to each strainer. After being plunged in liquid nitrogen, the cells cooled quickly, just as in vitrification with much larger electron microscope grids. After thawing, bulk-vitrified hES cells exhibited high survival rates—up to pproximately 94%. All surviving cell clumps generated hES cell colonies and showed pluripotency.

Another problem faced in cryopreservation by vitrification is the cytodamage produced by the cryoprotectant itself. With the vitrification approach, glass-like solidification of the freezing solution is achieved by using a high concentration of cryoprotectant and rapid cooling. Although this approach can eliminate cell injury due to ice crystal formation, the high concentration of cryoprotectant may induce significant toxic and osmotic damage. The concentrations of cryoprotectants required to achieve vitrification are inversely related to the rate of cooling. Therefore, an increased speed of cooling can lessen the cryoprotectant-induced toxicity, as it minimizes the time of exposure to these toxic compounds and allows their use at reduced concentrations.

Nishigaki et al. [73] developed a new cryoprotectant without DMSO, using a chemically defined DMSO-free and serum-free medium composed of Euro-Collins solution as a base medium and 40% EG and 10% polyethylene glycol (PEG) as cryoprotectants. When these cryoprotectants were employed in vitrification, the recovery ratio of hES cells was approximately 23%, compared with about 0.4% when the conventional slow freezing method was employed. The pluripotency of hES cells was maintained. The recovery rate was low compared with vitrification using tiny carriers, but the authors used 1.8 mL cryovials as Suemori et al. [11] instead of straws and strainers. The advantage of this method is easier handling compared with straw protocols. As described above, however, this method has many disadvantages.

5. Back to Slow Cooling Protocols

After an extensive search for optimal cryoprotocols for pluripotent stem cells, we returned to slow cooling protocols again, because these methods are very simple. Simple is best. The best way to overcome the various problems is to cryopreserve individual cells, not colony fragments. This is confirmed by the cryopreservation of mES cells. However, we must wait for the development of a suitable molecule before devising a new protocol. Krawetz et al. [74] wrote that one of the main drawbacks of the hES cell culture is that these cells are particularly sensitive to dissociation, which is required for passaging, expansion, cryopreservation, and other applications. Recently, an inhibitor of Rho kinase was discovered to increase the survival rate of single dissociated hES cells [75]. This breakthrough has allowed new methods in the hES cell culture to be developed, with the promise of increasing hES cell numbers to the realm of clinical relevance.

A. Ringleader of the Breakthrough–The Rock Inhibitor

The ROCK inhibitor Y-27632, (R)-(+)-*trans*-N-(4-pyridyl)-4-(1-aminoethyl)- cyclohexanecarboxamide 2HCl (formula: $C_{14}H_{21}N_3O$ 2HCl H_2O), has many important functions, regulating several types of gene pathways. The greatest advantage of Y-27632 in the field of ES cell and/or pluripotent stem cell cryopreservation is to permit a single ES cell to survive after complete dissociation. This is favorable for researchers struggling to overcome the various problems surrounding cryopreservation of hES and iPS cells. In 2008, two papers were published which proposed novel cooling protocols using Y-27632 [76,77], although these protocols differ to some extent. The authors indicate some problems, including slow freezing–rapid thawing and vitrification of colonies in suspension, poor and inconsistent viability, and high differentiation rates. However, their claims are not always justified because, as mentioned above, vitrification is relatively superior in terms of survival rate, and differentiation is not fatal. Even in conventional slow cooling protocols, with the use of new cryoprotectants survival rates are improved to some extent, although they are variable. What is required now is to cryopreserve a large number of hES cells with simple slow cooling protocols and to achieve high survival rates after thawing. The novel slow cooling method using Y-27632 is valuable because it fulfills both of these requirements and can supply intact hES cells in bulk for regenerative medicine. However, the authors of the two papers did not distinguish between the effects of freezing itself on cell survival rate and the effects of cell detachment and dissociation. Furthermore, although cell death is believed to be due to apoptosis, as mentioned above [7,13], what triggers apoptosis and whether other factors apart from apoptosis cause cell death is not known.

First, we consider the method developed by *Martin-Ibañez* et al. [76], who describe a protocol for cryopreserving completely dissociated single cells that has three components: (1) the use of the ROCK inhibitor Y-27632 in dissociation of the cells; (2) its addition to the freezing medium; (3) its addition to the culture medium after thawing. (1) 10μM Y-27632 is added to the culture medium 1 hour before detaching the cells from the feeder layer. Cells are enzymatically detached from this layer, followed by flushing with a pipette several times to detach single hES cells from the feeders. This treatment, however, masks the influence of freezing itself, because hES cells have been affected for 1 hour by the inhibitor and are frozen with the "memory" that they were immersed in the inhibitor. Therefore, if we try to estimate the influence of freezing itself on the cooling protocol using Y-27632, this treatment must be omitted or the inhibitor must be added to the freezing medium without immersion before freezing. (2) The freezing medium consists of 90% hES cell culture medium without bFGF supplemented with 10% DMSO and 10 μM Y-27632. Between 30,000 and 100,000 dissociated hESCs are loaded into a cryovial filled with the freezing medium and frozen at −1°C/minute to −80°C using a freezing container, and then stored in liquid nitrogen. (3) One to two weeks after cryopreservation, hES cells are rapidly thawed in a water bath set at 37°C, washed twice in hES cell culture medium, and plated on a fresh feeder layer. 10μM the ROCK inhibitor is added to this post-thawing medium. According to their results, the protecting effect of the ROCK inhibitor in the freezing medium on the cryopreserved single hES cells was approximately twice than in its absence, estimated by the Trypan Blue exclusion method.

Our data were not always identical to the authors' results, in which hES cell colonies were not immersed in before and during dissociation. Directly after thawing, the survival rate was 70–80% irrespective of the presence or absence of Y-27632. As time passed, cell death increased markedly in the post-thawing medium without Y-27632. Cell death did not occur immediately after dissociation and thawing. These processes will be referred to again later in this chapter.

The colony formation rate after thawing was highest in the presence of Y-27632 in both the freezing and post-thawing media, and was negligible in its absence from the post-thawing medium. From another point of view, however, their results appear perplexing because the final survival rate was below 1% based on the formation of 150–250 colonies from 30,000 hES cells. This value is the same as that obtained with the conventional cooling protocol, although in our data the survival rate was 9%–16% in the presence of Y-27632 in the post-thawing medium. The efficiency of colony formation was reduced by approximately five fold compared with that of dissociated hES cells in control conditions without cryopreservation. However, although these values are low, they are of more interest than those obtained with other protocols, because if 10^6 cells are frozen 10^4–10^5 colonies will be formed. It is useful to cryopreserve individual cells.

Martin-Ibañez et al. [76] attributed the low survival rate to differences among cell lines, variations between culture and cell passaging protocols, or overestimation of the number of alive hES cells counted after thawing by the Trypan Blue exclusion method. According to our previous data, the high survival rate irrespective of the use of the inhibitor immediately after thawing is not an overestimate: it is a true value. However, only a small number of colonies are formed in the medium containing Y-27632 despite using a large number of living single cells, though few colonies are found when Y-27632 is not added. Once cell death begins, it progresses continually. The inhibitor cannot completely suppress this powerful progressive process. Explanation of this relentless cell death march requires the hypothesis that hES cells attack themselves after thawing. This is a major theme of this chapter, and will be elaborated later in relation to DNA microarray analysis.

In this protocol the number of hES cells attached to the feeders was higher after thawing in the presence of the inhibitor compared with the control condition. This observation is suggestive, because adhesional molecules, particularly E-cadherins, are maintained by the ROCK inhibitor. Unexpected differentiation caused by this protocol is almost never detected.

In the same year as the publication of the work of Martin-Ibañez et al. [76], Li et al. [77] established another protocol using the ROCK inhibitor. The major difference from the protocol of *Martin-Ibañez* et al. [76] is the cryopreservation of small clumps rather than single cells. Their protocol is also very interesting because Y-27632 is effective in freezing not only single cells but also small amounts of tissue.

Other authors have modified this protocol. Xu et al. [78] proposed a new formula for a freezing solution containing 7.5% DMSO and 2.5% PEG in combination with the ROCK inhibitor and a p53 inhibitor, which enhanced ES cell recovery on the first day of culture by up to 30% compared with the freezing medium containing 10% DMSO and culture in the presence of the ROCK inhibitor; on the first day of post-thaw culture the presence of 10 μM Y-27632 and 1 μM pifithrin-mu together resulted in a further significant improvement in cell recovery of around 20%.

On the other hand, Bueno et al. [79] sounded a warning that we should heed. Although the use of cryopreserved cord blood (CB)-derived CD34+ hematopoietic stem and progenitor cells (HSPCs) leads to rapid hematopoietic recovery upon transplantation, current methods for ex vivo expansion of HSPCs continue to result in a loss of multilineage differentiation potential and current freeze-thawing protocols result in considerable cell death and loss of CD34+ HSPCs. The major cause of the loss of viability after slow freezing is apoptosis induced directly by cryoinjury. To suppress this apoptosis, CB-derived CD34+ HSPCs after MACS-isolation were treated with 10 μM of the inhibitor and were cryopreserved. They found that the inhibitor not only inhibited cell expansion of both fresh and cryopreserved CD34+ HSPCs but also impaired the survival/recovery of CD34+ HSPCs upon thawing regardless of whether the inhibitor was added to both the cryopreservation and the expansion medium or solely to the expansion medium. Their report suggests that this was because of differences in the effects of the inhibitor on human stem cells growing in suspension versus those growing attached to either treated tissue culture plastic or extracellular matrix.

B. What is the Mechanism of Cell Death Occurring in Cryopreserved Single hES Cells and its Suppression by the Rock Inhibitor?

As Heng et al. [13] indicated, cell death is predominantly caused by apoptosis instead of necrosis. Apoptosis is known to be the major mechanism that causes cell death. Apoptosis caused by cryopreservation has been reported by Park et al. [80], who indicated an increase in DNA fragmentation and apoptosis-related gene transcription, and a reduction in the developmental capacity of frozen–thawed embryos. Caspases play an important role in apoptotic processes [80]. Xu et al. [81] investigated how stimuli arising from cryopreservation result in apoptosis, which leads to low cell recovery rate after cryopreservation, and showed that caspases 8 and 9 are closely associated with apoptotic pathways. In addition, the level of reactive oxygen species is significantly increased and the F-actin content and distribution are altered. p53 is also activated and translocated into the nucleus. During cryopreservation, apoptosis is induced by activation of both caspases 8 and 9 through the extrinsic and intrinsic pathways, respectively. However, they emphasize that exactly how the extrinsic pathway is activated is still unclear and deserves further investigation. Moreover, the caspase inhibitor benzyloxycarbonyl-Val-Ala-DL-Asp-fluoromethylketone (Z-VAD-FMK) has been used in the cryopreservation of hES cells [83] to reduce apoptotic cell death. However, the idea of apoptosis following cryopreservation is outdated, because anybody hits upon it. If it is a single mechanism and true, this is good. Are any processes other than apoptosis concerned with cell death? Even if apoptotic processes play a major role in cell death, it is unknown why and how apoptosis starts. If we know what triggers apoptosis or how it begins, we may have another strategy to protect hES cells from cell death.

Li et al. [83] did not believe in the old-fashioned idea of apoptosis. They investigated the effects of Y-27632 on cell adhesion in cell adhesion assays. After single hES cells were cultured with or without 10 μM Y-27632 for 12 hrs, non-adherent cells were removed by gentle washing. Adherent cells were quantified using a fluorescence microplate reader at 494 nm excitation and 517 nm emission wavelengths. When the medium was supplemented with 10 μM of the inhibitor, small cell aggregates formed and viability increased. The aggregates were tight, spherical, and smooth, and were dissociated into single cells by treatment with EGTA and gentle pipetting.

Analysis of apoptosis showed that 80% of cells were viable after dissociation and 66% of thawed hES cells were viable. When regularly passaged hES cells were dissociated into single cells and immediately subjected to apoptosis analysis, a small percentage of cells were dead and/or apoptotic. When these dissociated single cells were cryopreserved in liquid nitrogen, thawed, and then immediately subjected to apoptosis analysis, an increase in cell mortality was observed; however, these results indicate that only a small percentage of cells died as a result of cryopreservation. From these curious phenomena, Li et al. [83] proposed the following hypothesis. As Y-27632 transduces signals from the cortical actin cytoskeleton and ECM to the nucleus, leading to changes in cell morphology as well as transcriptional regulation, by interrupting signals from the cellular environment by inhibiting ROCK, hES cells lose their sensitivity to the current environment. Therefore, hES cells treated with Y-27632 are no longer able to detect that they have been dissociated into single cells and cannot assess the current state of the plasma membrane or actin cytoskeleton during/after cryopreservation. In effect, the inhibitor does not block apoptotic pathways but, more accurately, causes hES cells to become “blind”, “deaf,” and “dumb” with respect to their current environment. This ignorance allows hES cells to aggregate into small colonies and this cell–cell interaction is responsible for the reduction in apoptosis observed in the inhibitor-treated groups. That the cell death observed after thawing is not completely due to apoptosis is an attractive proposition. However, this hypothesis has little supporting evidence.

Cell death after thawing is characterized as follows: (1) cell death does not stop but continues for some time; (2) hES cells after thawing adhere neither to the plate nor to each other.

Because cell death continues, it is reasonable to expect that a continuous self-offensive mechanism is established. Furthermore, it is natural that prompt or smooth cell-to-cell re-adhesion is concerned with the maintenance and distribution of adhesional molecules. As mentioned above, E-cadherin is the most promising candidate.

First, we will consider why cell death continues and the self-offensive mechanism that promotes this process. One way to solve a difficult problem in the absence of clues is to have a tool with many capabilities, even though the information it provides may be complicated. Gene pathway analysis is best suited for this purpose. The experimental design was as follows.

hES cell colonies were partially dissociated into clumps. Next, after removing MEF cells, hES cell clumps were incubated in 0.25% trypsin–EDTA at 37°C for 4 minutes, pipetted in either conditioned medium containing 10 μM of the ROCK inhibitor or control medium without the ROCK inhibitor, dissociated, and transferred to cryovials filled with 1 mL freezing medium consisting of the hES cell culture medium with 10% DMSO, and frozen slowly in a freezing container to −80°C overnight. The cooling rate of the Bicell was as described in our previous report [50]. The dissociated cells were stored in liquid nitrogen for more than 1 week and then rapidly thawed in a water bath set at 37°C.

Four different experimental conditions were used to investigate the effect of the ROCK inhibitor on cryopreserved dissociated hES cells: addition of 10 μM Y-27632 to the freezing medium and post-thawing medium (condition * 1); addition of 10 μM Y-27632 only to the freezing solution (*2); addition only to the post-thawing medium (* 3); and no addition to any medium (* 4). After thawing, the ROCK inhibitor-treated hES cells were alive; they adhered to the plate readily as single cells, and proliferated (Fig. 5).

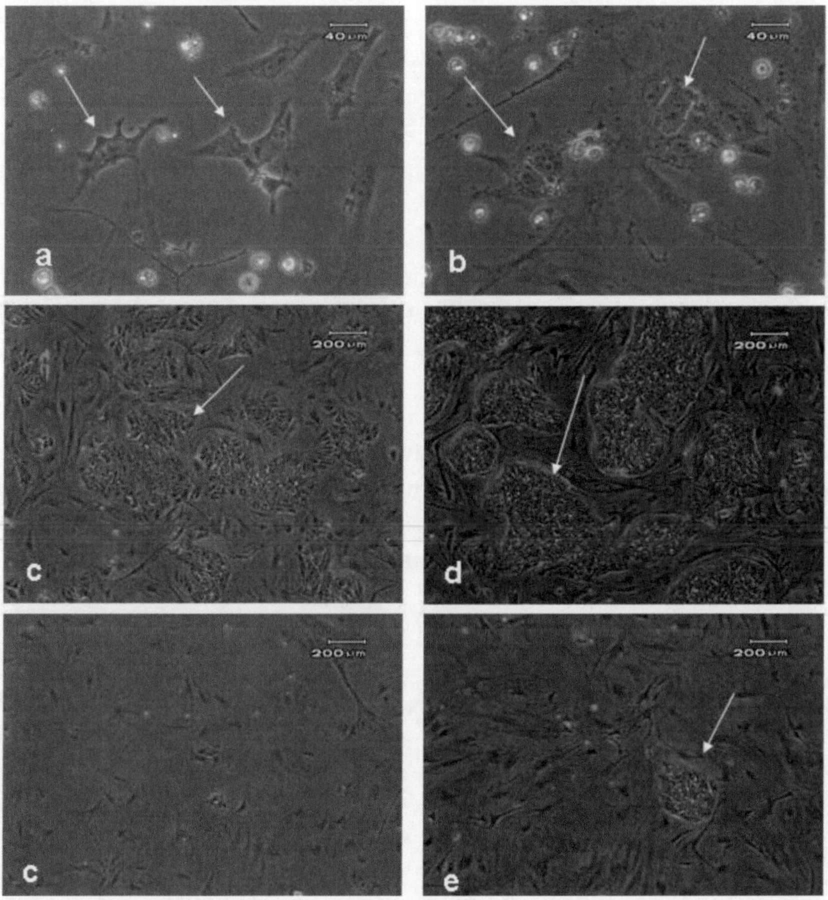

Figure5. a. hES cells treated by the ROCK inhibitor Y-27632 (arrows in the condition *1) adhere to the plate as a single cell , then and extend. b. They proliferate at day 1 after thawing. c. A large number of colonies appear at day 2. d. At day 5 after thawing, colonies are sufficiently large to prepare for cell passage. e. Almost no live cells are found among the untreated hES cells (condition *4). f. At day 5, a few small colonies can be seen.

To estimate the survival rate, 300 cells were cultured under each condition for 10 days. The number of colonies was divided by 300. The survival rates were approximately 17%(condition *1), 1%(*2), 9%(*3), and 0.5%(*4). From these data, the treated hES cells (*1) showed a high rate of survival, 35 times higher than the untreated group (*4). Addition of the inhibitor to the medium after thawing (*1&*3) is more effective. In addition to dissociation, cryopreservation itself promotes cell death.

To understand the mechanism of cell death, especially how it is initiated and why it progresses with time, DNA microarray analysis was performed. Total RNA of cells from each condition (*1, *2, *3 and *4) was extractedand was treated according to Yamamoto et al. [84]. The reacted chips were scanned using a DNA microarray scanner. The intensity values of each feature of the scanned image were quantified using an analysis software. Expression ratios were calculated for features that were present in both reference (*1) and tested samples(*2, *3, *4). GENMAP version 2.1 (http://www.genmapp.org) analysis was performed using gene database Hs-Std_20060526.gdb [85,86]. The microarray data was deposited into NCBI GEO with accession number GSE21796, (http://www.ncbi.nlm.nih.gov/geo/query/acc.cgi?acc=GSE21796).

Table 1. Log ratio of experimental samples (conditions *2, *3, *4) versus the reference sample (condition *1) at 12hours after thawing. Between *3 and *1, few differences were observed, but some differences (gray boxes) are perceived in *2 & *4 containing the ROCK inhibiter Y-27632 comparing with *1

GeneID	Symbol	*2(vs*1)	*3(vs*1)	*4(vs*1)
843	CASP10	0.66	0.08	0.33
841	CASP8	0.88	0.14	0.84
836	CASP3	-0.26	-0.35	-0.66
130399	ACVR1C	0.74	0.18	0.89
3553	IL1B	0.03	0.17	0.57
3554	IL1R1	0.3	0.25	1.04
7040	TGFB1	0.51	0.19	0.34
7043	TGFB3	0.92	-0.13	0.82
397	ARHGDIB	2.09	-0.01	2.31
998	CDC42	0.68	-0.17	0.56
5879	RAC1	0.17	0.34	-0.38

Cell death increased for 12 hours after thawing, and then plateaued. From DNA microarray analysis of the apoptosis-associated genes, caspases 8 and 10 were upregulated in *2 compared to that in *1 (Table). In *4, caspase 8 was upregulated compared with*1. In the absence of Y-27632 in the post-thawing medium, apoptosis was induced through caspases 8 and 10; this theory is supported by Xu et al. [81] although in their report caspases 8 and 9, and not caspase 10, were activated after cryopreservation. Caspases 8 and 10 are initiator caspases [87]. Executioner caspases (caspases 3 and 7) remain inactive for at least at 12 hours after thawing, though caspase 8 and/or 10 are known to be required for caspase 3 activation [88]. Another feature of caspases 8 and 10 is their association with the extrinsic pathway.

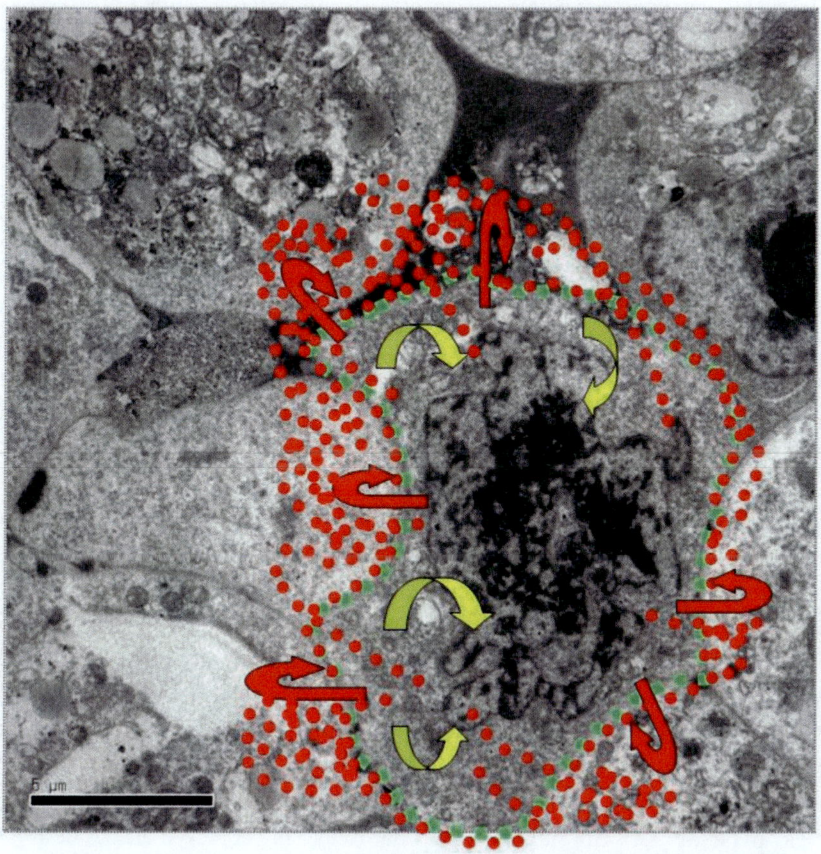

Figure 6. The scheme of apoptotic trigger mapping to the electron micrographic image in which with the apoptotic events e.g. fragmentation of nucleus is found at 2 hours after thawing. It shows IL-1 and/or TGF-beta (red dots) are produced and released from the cell, turn over (red arrows) and react against their receptors (pale green squares) expressed on the membrane, which activate caspase family (yellow arrows).

As Xu et al. [80] suggested, however, the way in which the extrinsic pathway is activated remains unknown. Through this DNA microarray analysis, we began to understand what triggers the activation of caspase 8. As seen in the Table, TGF-β and IL-1β and their respective receptors, ACVR1C and IL-1R, were upregulated in *4 compared with *1. No difference was observed between the experimental sample (*3) and the reference sample (*1). According to human gene information data (Hs-Std_20060526.gdb) and human pathway data (Hs_Contributed_20070308) provided by the Gene Map Annotator and Pathway Profile (http://www.genmapp.org), the initiator caspases, i.e., caspases 8 and 10 are components of the mitogen-activated protein kinase (MAPK) signaling complex and can be activated through the TGF-β and the IL-1β pathways [85,86]. Interestingly, activation of IL-1β and its receptor are lost in *2 i.e., the freezing medium containing the ROCK inhibitor Y-27632, and only one route through the TGF-β enhances caspase 8. This difference may reflect apoptosis due to dissociation.We now have an answer to the question what triggers the apoptotic process. It is a cytokine storm. Stem cells are very finicky when they come under stress, and they usually kill themselves [68]. Under severe stress, single hES cells produce TGF-β and/or IL-1β, receive stimuli through enhanced receptors, upregulate caspase 8, and progress to apoptosis. This cytokine storm is partly suppressed by the ROCK inhibitor. Other methods of blocking cytokines or their receptors may well increase the survival rate. Figure 6 shows a schematic representation of this mechanism.

It is difficult to completely explain cell death in terms of apoptosis. Apoptosis accounted only for a small proportion of cell death in a flow cytometry study by the TUNEL method [83]. From DNA microarray analysis, we found another cell death mechanism associated with disarray of actin filaments. ARHGDIB and Cdc42, subcomponents of the G13 signaling pathway, were upregulated in conditions *2&*4 compared with *1 (Table). This pathway passes through ARHGDIB and Cdc42 by RhoA activation and re-organizes actin filaments [89,90]. Cdc42 directly affects actin remodeling and function [91,92]. *Arhgdib* is a component of the G13 gene pathway and its activation in turn activates *Cdc* and *Rac* [93]. Hyperactivation of this pathway causes disarray of filaments. This pathway is closely associated with intercellular junctions, especially adherence junctions, because adherence junctions are constructed from cadherin family members and are affected by cytoplasmic actin filaments through anchor proteins, such as catenin [94]. The expression of E-cadherins is markedly higher in undifferentiated cells and their distribution is relatively homogeneous in hES cells [34]. Other research has shown that a higher E-cadherin level is associated with a higher likelihood of agglomeration and subsequent survival in suspension [35]. As Singh et al. [35] noted, E-cadherin level is maintained in the ROCK inhibitor-treated hES cells, which rapidly form colonies consisting of five to ten hES cells before proliferation and are revived again. Without the ROCK inhibitor treatment, however, single hES cells do not form colonies and do not survive. Intramembrane proteins aggregate and become distributed on one side of the membrane after thawing as time passes. According to Popoff and Geny [94], Rac and Cdc42 mainly coordinate the assembly and disassembly of adherence junctional components. Moreover, a subtle balance of Rho/Ras-GTPase activity and interplay between these molecules is required to maintain optimal organization and function of junctions. Lin et al. [95] showed that in zebrafish, Galpha(12/13) regulates epiboly, a cell movement seen in the early embryo, in part by associating with the cytoplasmic terminus of E-cadherins, and thereby inhibiting E-cadherin activity and cell adhesion; they demonstrated that Galpha(12/13) modulates epibolic movements of the enveloping layer by regulating actin cytoskeleton organization through a RhoGEF/Rho-dependent pathway. From these findings, we conclude that hyperactivation of the G13 signaling pathway after thawing disrupts the functional balance between the actin cytoskeletal system and E-cadherins, deforms cell shape; inhibits adhesion to other cells, does not re-establish cooperation among cells, and guides individual hES cells toward cell death. The march toward cell death is suppressed, but not completely, by the ROCK inhibitor—the survival rate is only 17%. Cell death pathways other than MAPK and G13 signaling pathways will need to be considered in future.

6. What Cryopreservation Methods are Used for hiPS Cells?

hiPS cells are similar to hES cells in morphology, proliferation, surface antigens, gene expression, epigenetic status of pluripotent cell-specific genes, karyotypes, and telomerase activity [2,96]. The cryoprotocols established in hES cells are therefore applied to hiPS cells and, as expected, are effective.

Holm et al. [97] froze iPS cells as single-cell suspensions with the ROCK inhibitor Y-27632 and the novel freezing medium containing 10% DMSO, glucose, and a high polymer in addition to NaCl, KCl, Na_2HPO_4, HK_2PO_4, and $NaHCO_3$ in the freezing container, and then stored in a liquid nitrogen tank.

The cells were re-suspended in 1 mL SR containing Y-27632 diluted 1:500. The authors have not stated the duration of the presence of Y-27632 in the culture medium after thawing. They compared the novel freezing medium with the SR medium containing 10% DMSO. After thawing, the cells had a high level of viability (90%–96%) in the former without any impact on proliferation and differentiation compared with the latter (49%). The colony formation rate of hES cells of the former was more than three times that of the latter. In iPS cells, it was 100% (500,000/500,000) in the former. The survival rate, however, of the control was extremely good. Beside any superiority of the novel freezing medium, the good results in the control may be due to the cell lines used. For example, in our data the survival rates immediately after thawing were 81%–87% in *1&*3 conditions and 68%–79% in *2&*4 of both hES cell lines, but 66%–70% in *1&*3 and 60%–63% in *2&*4 of one iPS cell line. The survival rate of iPS cells was clearly lower than that of hES cells.

Recent papers [97,98,99] have reported the use of cryoprotocols using Y-27632 in iPS cells. *Claassen*_et al. [99] froze cells in a freezing medium containing 20% DMSO and cultured them in a thawing medium containing 10 μM Y-27632. The number of colonies was seven times higher than that in the control. In ES cells a four-fold increase was observed. *Baharvand* et al. [98] reported that the addition of the ROCK inhibitor to both pre- and post-thaw culture media increased cloning efficiency. The presence of Y-27632 in Matrigel further increased cloning efficiency.

Conclusion

Although cryoprotocols for human pluripotent stem cells have changed considerably since 1998, they began as slow cooling protocols and have now returned to slow cooling protocols. This is appropriate, because these techniques are simple and can cope with the bulk freezing necessary for regenerative medicine. But there are still some problems to overcome. The mechanisms of cell death are not completely understood. There may be pathways other than those mentioned in this chapter that remain to be elucidated. Existing protocols will be further improved and new ones will be devised. Cryoprotectants still have some toxicity, and it is important to reduce their toxicity, especially for slow cooling protocols. Bulk cryopreservation requires a new device. Cryoprotocols have not yet been established for various stem cell-derived cells, but these will inevitably be required and developed in future. Some differentiated cell types resist freezing, but others are easily frozen. Differentiated target cells show little resistance to freezing, but immature target cells do not always show the same behavior on freezing as differentiated cells. Pluripotent stem cells offer considerable scope for overcoming the difficulty of cryopreservation in some cell types because they can be used to supply various cell types, from immature to mature stages.

Acknowledgments

We thank Mr. Ken Matsumoto of Nissui Pharmaceutical Co. for providing the culture medium and Mr. Naohiro Nakata and Youichi Abo, Air Water, Inc. for allowing us to use the programmable freezer. We also thank Mr. Susumu Ito, Ms. Kayo Suzuki, and Dr. Kiyokazu Kametani of the Research Center for Instrumental Analysis, Shinshu University, for their excellent technical assistance.

References

[1] Thomson, J.A., Itskovitz-Eldor, J., Shapiro, S.S., Waknitz, M.A., Swiergiel, J.J., Marshall, V.S., & Jones, J.M.(1998). Embryonic stem cell lines derived from human blastocysts. *Science*. 282:1145-1147.

[2] Takahashi, K., Tanabe, K., Ohnuki, M., Narita, M., Ichisaka, T., Tomoda, K., & Yamanaka, S. (2007). Induction of pluripotent stem cells from adult human fibroblasts by defined factors. *Cell*. 131:861-872.

[3] Mazur, P.(1970). Cryobiology: The freezing of biological systems. *Science*. 168:939-949.

[4] Pegg, D.E. (2007). Principles of cryopreservation. *Method Mol Biol.* 368:39-57.

[5] Polge, C., Smith, A.U., & Parkes, A.S.(1940). Revival of spermatozoa after vitrification and dehydration at low temperature. *Nature* 164:666.

[6] Murdoch, L.(1982). Dimethyl sulfoxide (DMSO)--an overview. *Can J Hosp Pharm*. 35:79-85.

[7] Heng, B.C., Kuleshova, L.L., Bested, S.M., Liu, H., & Cao, T.(2005). The cryopreservation of human embryonic stem cells. *Biotechnol Appl Biochem*. 41:97-104.

[8] Johkura, K., Cui, L., Asanuma, K., Okouchi, Y., Ogiwara, N., & Sasaki, K.(2004). Cytochemical and ultrastructural characterization of growing colonies of human embryonic stem cells. *J Anat* 205:247-255.

[9] Reubinoff, B.E., Pera, M.F., Vajta, G., & Trounson, A.O.(2001). Effective cryopreservation of human embryonic stem cells by the open pulled straw vitrification method. *Hum Reprod.* 16:2187-2194.

[10] Richards, M., Fong, C.Y., Tan, S., Chan, W.K., & Bongso, A.(2004). An efficient and safe xeno-free cryopreservation method for the storage of human embryonic stem cells. *Stem Cells.* 22:779-89.

[11] Suemori, H., Yasuchika, K., Hasegawa, K., Fujioka, T., Tsuneyoshi, N., & Nakatsuj, N.(2006). Efficient establishment of human embryonic stem cell lines and long-term maintenance with stable karyotype by enzymatic bulk passage. *Biochem Biophys Res Commun.* 345:926-932.

[12] Li, Y., Tan, J.C., & Li, L.S.(2010). Comparison of three methods for cryopreservation of human embryonic stem cells. *Fertil Steril.* 93:999-1005.

[13] Heng, B.C., Ye, C.P., Liu, H., Toh, W.S., Rufaihah, A.J., Yang, Z., Bay, B.H., Ge, Z., Ouyang, H.W., Lee, E.H., & Cao, T.J.(2006). Loss of viability during freeze-thaw of intact and adherent human 13:433-445.

[14] Kent, L.(2009). Freezing and thawing human embryonic stem cells. *J Vis Exp.* 24; pii: 1555. doi: 10.3791/1555.

[15] Katkov, I.I., Kim, M.S., Bajpai, R., Altman, Y.S., Mercola, M., Loring, J.F., Terskikh, A.V., Snyder, E.Y., & Levine, F.(2006). Cryopreservation by slow cooling with DMSO diminished production of Oct-4 pluripotency marker in human embryonic stem cells. *Cryobiology.* 53:194-205.

[16] Ha, S.Y., Jee, B.C., Suh, C.S., Kim, H.S., Oh, S.K., Kim, S.H., & Moon.(2005). Cryopreservation of human embryonic stem cells without the use of a programmable freezer. *Hum Reprod.* 20:1779-1785.

[17] Miyamoto, H., & Ishibashi, T.J.(1977). Survival of frozen-thawed mouse and rat embryos in the presence of ethylene 50:373-375.

[18] Sola-Penna, M., & Meyer-Fernandes, J.R.(1998). Stabilization against thermal inactivation promoted by sugars on enzyme structure and function: why is trehalose more effective than other sugars? *Arch Biochem Biophys.* 360:10-14.

[19] Wu, C.F., Tsung, H.C., Zhang, W.J., Wang, Y., Lu J.H., Tang, Z.Y., Kuang, Y.P., Jin, W., Cui, L., Liu, W., & Cao, Y.L.(2005). Improved cryopreservation of human embryonic stem cells with trehalose. *Reprod Biomed Online.*11:733-739.

[20] Kim, S.J., Park, J.H., Lee, J.E., Kim, J.M., Lee, J.B., Moon., Roh, S.I., Kim, C.G., & Yoon, H.S.(2004). *Stem Cells. Effects of type IV collagen and laminin on the cryopreservation of human embryonic stem cells.* 22:950-961.

[21] Ji, L., de Pablo, J.J., & Palecek, S.P.(2004). Cryopreservation of adherent human embryonic stem cells. *Biotechnol Bioeng.* 88:299-312.

[22] Amit, M., Carpenter, M.K., Inokuma, M.S., Chiu, C.P., Harris, C.P., Waknitz, M.A., Itskovitz-Eldor, J., & Thomson, J.A.(2000). Clonally derived human embryonic stem cell lines maintain pluripotency and proliferative potential for prolonged periods of culture. *Dev Biol.* 227:271-278.

[23] Reubinoff, B.E., Pera, M.F., Fong, C.Y., Trounson, A., & Bongso, A.(2000). Embryonic stem cell lines from human blastocysts: somatic differentiation in vitro. *Nat Biotechnol.* 18:399-404.

[24] Sathananthan, H., Pera, M., & Trounson, A.(2002). The fine structure of human embryonic stem cells. *Reprod Biomed Online.* 4:56-61.

[25] Yang, P.F., Hua, T.C., Wu, J., Chang, Z.H., Tsung, H.C., & Cao, Y.L.(2006). Cryopreservation of human embryonic stem cells: A protocol by programmed cooling. *CryoLetters.* 27:361-368.

[26] Huettner, J.E., Lu, A., Qu, Y., Wu, Y., Kim, M., & McDonald, J.W. (2006). Gap junctions and connexon hemichannels in human *Stem Cells.* 24:1654-1667.

[27] Wong, R.C., Pébay, A., Nguyen, L.T., Koh, K.L., & Pera, M.F.(2004). Presence of functional gap junctions in human *Stem Cells.* 22:883-889.

[28] Wolvetang, E.J., Pera, M.F., & Zuckerman, K.S.(2007). Gap junction mediated transport *Biochem Biophys Res Commun.* 363:610-615.

[29] Wong, R.C., Pébay, A., Nguyen, L.T., Koh, K.L., & Pera, M.F.(2004). Presence of functional gap junctions in human *Stem Cells.* 22:883-889.

[30] Wong, R.C., Dottori, M., Koh, K.L., Nguyen, L.T., Pera, M.F., & Pébay, A.(2006). Gap junctions modulate apoptosis *Biochem Biophys Res Commun.* 344:181-188.

[31] Wong, R.C., & Pébay, A.(2010). Study of gap junctions in human *Methods Mol Biol.* 584:211-228.

[32] Van Hoof, D., Braam, S.R., Dormeyer, W., Ward-van Oostwaard, D., Heck, A.J., Krijgsveld, J.,& Mummery, C.L.(2008). Feeder-free monolayer *Stem Cells.* 26:2777-2781.

[33] Spencer, H., Keramari, M., & Ward, C.M.(2011).Using cadherin expression to assess spontaneous differentiation of embryonic stem cells. *Methods Mol Biol.* 690:81-94.

[34] Li, Z., Qiu, D., Sridharan, I., Qian, X., Zhang, H., Zhang, C., & Wang, R.(2010). Spatially resolved quantification of E-cadherin on target hES cells. *J Phys Chem B.* 114:2894-2900.

[35] Singh, H., Mok, P., Balakrishnan, T., Rahmat, S.N., & Zweigerdt, R.(2010). Up-scaling single cell-inoculated suspension culture of human embryonic stem cells. *Stem Cell Res.* 4:165-179.

[36] Li, L., Wang, S., Jezierski, A., Moalim-Nour, L., Mohib, K., Parks, R.J., Retta, S.F., & Wang, L. (2010). Individual cell movement, asymmetric colony expansion, rho-associated kinase, and E-cadherin impact the clonogenicity of human embryonic stem cells. unique interplay between Rap1 and E-cadherin in the endocytic pathway regulates self-renewal of human embryonic stem cells. *Stem Cells.* 28:247-257.

[37] Li, L., Wang, B.H., Wang, S., Moalim-Nour, L., Mohib, K., Lohnes, D., & Wang, L. (2010). Individual cell movement, asymmetric colony expansion, rho-associated kinase, and E-cadherin impact the clonogenicity of human embryonic stem cells. *Biophys J.* 98:2442-2451.

[38] Chen, G., Hou, Z., Gulbranson, D.R., & Thomson, J.A.(2010). Actin-myosin contractility is responsible for the reduced viability of dissociated human embryonic stem cells. *Cell Stem Cell.* 7:240-248.

[39] Ohgushi, M., Matsumura, M., Eiraku, M., Murakami, K., Aramaki, T., Nishiyama, A., Muguruma, K., Nakano, T., Suga, H., Ueno, M., Ishizaki, T., Suemori, H., Narumiya, S., Niwa, H., & Sasai Y.(2010). Molecular pathway and cell state responsible for dissociation-induced apoptosis in human pluripotent stem cells. *Cell Stem Cell.* 7:225-239.

[40] Li, D., Zhou, J., Wang, L., Shin, ME., Su, P., Lei, X., Kuang, H., Guo, W., Yang, H., Cheng, L., Tanaka, T.S., Leckband, D.E., Reynolds, A.B., Duan, E., & Wang, F.(2010). Integrated biochemical and mechanical signals regulate multifaceted human embryonic stem cell functions. *J Cell Biol.* 191:631-644.

[41] Walker, A., Su, H., Conti, M.A., Harb, N., Adelstein, R.S., & Sato, N.(2010). Non-muscle myosin II regulates survival threshold of pluripotent stem cells. *Nat.Commun. 1(6):doi:10.1038/ncomms*1074, 2010.

[42] Zvibel, I., Smets, F., & Soriano, H.(2002). Anoikis: roadblock to cell transplantation? *Cell Transplant.* 11:621-630.

[43] Maruyama, M., Kenmochi, T., Sakamoto, K., Arita, S., Iwashita, C., & Kashiwabara, H. (2004). Simplified method for cryopreservation of islets using hydroxyethyl starch and dimethyl sulfoxide as cryoprotectants. *Transplant Proc.* 36:1133-1134.

[44] Richards, M., Fong, C.Y., Tan, S., Chan, W.K., & Bongso, A. (2005). An efficient and safe xeno-free cryopreservation *Stem Cells*. 22:779-789.

[45] Yang, P.F., Hua, T.C., Tsung, H.C., Cheng, Q.K., & Cao, Y.L.(2005). Effective cryopreservation *Conf Proc IEEE Eng Med Biol Soc*. 1:482-485.

[46] Yang, P.F., Hua, T.C., Wu, J., Chang, Z.H., Tsung, H.C., & Cao, Y.L. (2006). Cryopreservation of human *Cryo Letters*. 27:361-368.

[47] Ware, C.B., Nelson, A.M., & Blau, C.A. (2005). Controlled-rate freezing *Biotechniques*. 38:879-880; 882-883.

[48] Ware, C.B. & Baran, S.W.(2007). A controlled-cooling protocol for cryopreservation of human and non-human primate embryonic stem cells. *Methods Mol Biol*. 407:43-49.

[49] Lee J.Y., Lee J.E., Kim D.K., Yoon T.K., Chung H.M., & Lee D.R.(2010). High concentration of synthetic serum, stepwise equilibration and slow cooling as an efficient technique for large-scale cryopreservation of human embryonic stem cells. *Fertil Steril*. 93:976-985.

[50] Ichikawa, H., No, H., Takei, S., Takashimizu, I., Yue, F., Cui, L., Ogiwara, N., Johkura, K., Nishimoto, Y., & Sasaki, K.(2007). Cryopreservation of mouse embryoid bodies. *Cryobiology*. 54:290-293.

[51] Li, Y., Tan, J.C., & Li, L.S.(2010). Comparison of three methods for cryopreservation of human embryonic stem cells. *Fertil Steril*. 93:999-1005.

[52] Debenedetti, P.G., & Stanley, H.E.(2003). Supercooled and glassy water. *Physics Today* 56:40-46.

[53] Vajta, G., Holm, P., Kuwayama, M., Booth, P.J., Jacobsen, H., Greve, T., & Callesen, H. (1998). Open Pulled Straw (OPS) vitrification: a new way to reduce cryoinjuries of bovine ova and embryos. *Mol Reprod Dev*. 51:53-58.

[54] Moor, H., & Mühlethaler, K. (1963). Fine structure in frozen-etched yeast cells. *J Cell Biol*. 17:609-628.

[55] Heuser, J.E., Reese, T.S., & Landis, D.M. (1976). Preservation of synaptic structure *Cold Spring Harb Symp Quant Biol*. 40:17-24.

[56] Ichikawa, A., Ichikawa, M., & Sasaki, K. (1989) Freeze-substitution *J Electron Microsc*. 38:S118-122.

[57] Ichikawa, A., Ichikawa, M., &Hirokawa, N.(1980). The ultrastructure *Am J Anat*. 157:107-110.

[58] Ichikawa, M., Sasaki, K., & Ichikawa, A. (1989). Immunocytochemical localization *J Histochem Cytochem*. 37:185-94.

[59] Ichikawa, M., Sasaki, K., & Ichikawa, A.(1989). Optimal preparatory procedures of cryofixation for immunocytochemistry. *J Electron Microsc Tech*. 12:88-94.
[60] Bald, W.B.(1983). Optimizing the cooling *J Microsc*. 131(Pt 1):11-23.
[61] Ichikawa, M., & Ichikawa, A.(1987). The fine structure *Cell Tissue Res*. 250:305-314.
[62] Pegg, D.E.(2002). The history and principles of cryopreservation. *Seminars in reproductive medicine* 20:5-13.
[63] Elford, B.C., & Walter, C.A.(1972). Effects of electrolyte composition and pH on the structure and function of smooth muscle cooled to-79°C in Unfrozen media. *Cryobiology*. 9:82-100.
[64] Reubinoff, B.E., Pera, M.F., Vajta, G., & Trounson, A.O.(2001). Effective cryopreservation of human embryonic stem cells by the open pulled straw vitrification method. *Hum Reprod*. 16(10):2187-9214.
[65] Zhou, C.Q., Mai Q.Y., Li, T., & Zhuang, G.L.(2004). Cryopreservation of human *Chin Med J*. 117:1050-1055.
[66] Tedder, R.S., Zuckerman, M.A., Goldstone, A.H., Hawkins, A.E., Fielding, A., Briggs, E.M., Irwin, D., Blair, S., Gorman, A.M., Patterson, K.G.,Limch,D.C., Heptonstall,J.,&Brink,N.S. (1995). Hepatitis B transmission from contaminated cryopreservation tank. *Lancet*, 346, 137-140.
[67] Fujioka, T., Yasuchika, K., Nakamura, Y., Nakatsuji, N., & Suemori, H.(2004). A simple and efficient cryopreservation method for primate embryonic stem cells. *Int J Dev Biol*. 48:1149-1154.
[68] Brumfiel, G.(2004). Cell Biology: just add water. *Nature*. 428:14-15.
[69] Martino, A., Songasen, N., & Leibo, S.P.(1996). Development into blastocysts of bovine oocyte cryopreserved by ultra-rapid cooling. *Biol. Reprod*. 54: 1059-1069.
[70] Mavrides, A., & Morroll, D.(2002). Cryopreservation of bovine oocytes: is cryoloop vitrification the future to preserving the female gamete? *Reprod Nutr Dev*. 42:73-80.
[71] Lane, M., Schoolcraft, W.B. and Gardner, D.K.(1999). Vitrification of mouse and human blastocysts using a novel cryoloop container-less technique. *Fertil Steril*. 72:1073-1078.
[72] Li, T., Zhou, C., Liu, C., Mai, Q., & Zhuang, G.(2008). Bulk vitrification of human embryonic stem cells. *Hum Reprod*. 23:358-364.
[73] Nishigaki, T., Teramura, Y., Suemori, H., & Iwata, H.(2010). Cryopreservation of primate 60:159-164.

[74] Krawetz, R.J., Li, X., & Rancourt, D.E. (2009). Human embryonic stem cells: caught between a ROCK inhibitor and a hard place. Bioessays. 31:336-343.

[75] Watanabe, K., Ueno, M., Kamiya, D., Nishiyama, A., Matsumura, M., Wataya, T., Takahashi, J.B., Nishikawa, S., Nishikawa, S., Muguruma, K., Sasai, Y. (2007). A ROCK inhibitor permits survival of dissociated human embryonic stem cells. *Nat. Biotechnol.* 25, 681-686.

[76] Martin-Ibañez, R., Unger, C., Strömberg, A., Baker, D., Canals, J.M., & Hovatta, O.(2008). Novel cryopreservation method for dissociated human embryonic stem cells in the presence of a ROCK inhibitor. *Hum Reprod.* 23:2744-2754.

[77] Li, X., Meng, G., Krawetz, R., Liu, S., & Rancourt, D.E.(2008). The ROCK inhibitor Y-27632 enhances the survival rate of human embryonic stem cells following cryopreservation. *Stem Cells Dev.* 17:1079-1085.

[78] Xu, X., Cowley, S., Flaim, C.J., James, W., Seymour, L.W., & Cui, Z.(2010). Enhancement of cell recovery for dissociated human embryonic stem cells after cryopreservation. *Biotechnol Prog.* 26:781-788.

[79] Bueno, C., Montes, R., & Menendez, P. (2010). The ROCK inhibitor Y-27632 negatively affects the expansion/survival of both fresh and cryopreserved cord blood-derived CD34+ hematopoietic progenitor cells: Y-27632 negatively affects the expansion/survival of CD34+HSPCs. *Stem Cell Rev.* 6:215-223.

[80] Park, S.Y., Kim, E.Y., Cui, X.S., Tae, J.C., Lee, W.D, Kim, N.H., Park, S.P., Lim, J.H.(2006). Increase in DNA fragmentation and apoptosis-related gene expression in frozen-thawed bovine blastocysts. *Zygote* 4:125-131.

[81] Xu, X., Cowley. S., Flaim, C.J., James, W., Seymour, L., & Cui Z.(2010). The roles of apoptotic pathways in the low recovery rate after cryopreservation of dissociated human embryonic stem cells. *Biotechnol Prog.* 26:827-837.

[82] Heng, B.C., Clement, M.V., & Cao, T.(2007). Caspase inhibitor Z-VAD-FMK enhances the freeze-thaw survival rate of human embryonic stem cells. *Biosci Rep.* 27:257-264.

[83] Li, X., Krawetz, R., Liu, S., Meng, G., & Rancourt, D.E.(2009). ROCK inhibitor improves survival of cryopreserved serum/feeder-free single human embryonic stem cells. *Hum Reprod.* 24:580-589.

[84] Yamamoto, Y., Banas, A., Murata, S., Ishikawa, M., Lim CR, Teratani, T., Hatada, I., Matsubara, K., Kato, T., & Ochiya, T.(2008). A comparative analysis of the transcriptome and signal pathways in hepatic differentiation of human adipose mesenchymal stem cells. *FEBS J* 275:1260-1273.

[85] Doniger, S.W., Salomonis, N., Dahlquist, K.D., Vranizan, K., Lawlor, S.C., & Conklin, B.R.(2003). MAPPFinder: using Gene Ontology and GenMAPP to create a global gene-expression profile from microarray data. *Genome Biol.* 4:R7.

[86] Dahlquist, K.D., Salomonis, N., Vranizan, K., Lawlor, S.C.,& Conklin, B.R.(2002). GenMAPP, a new tool for viewing and analyzing microarray data on biological pathways. *Nat Genet.* 31:19-20.

[87] Boatright, K.M., & Salvesen, G.S.(2003). Mechanisms of caspase activation. *Curr Opin Cell Biol.* 15:725-231.

[88] Lai, J.M., Hsieh, C.L., & Chang, Z.F.(2003). Caspase activation during phorbol ester-induced apoptosis requires ROCK-dependent myosin-mediated contraction. *J Cell Sci* 116:3491-3501.

[89] Maekawa, M., Ishizaki, T., Boku,,S., Watanabe, N., Fujita,A., Iwamatsu,A., Obinata,T.,Ohashi,K., Mizuno,K., & Marumiya,S. (1999). Signaling from Rho to the actin cytoskeleton through protein kinases ROCK and LIM-kinase, *Science* 285: 895-898.

[90] Neves, S.R., Ram, P.T., & Iyengar, R.(2002). G protein pathways. *Science*. 296:1636-1639.

[91] Gerthoffer, W.T.(2005). Actin cytoskeletal dynamics in smooth muscle contraction. *Can J Physiol Pharmacol.* 83:851-856.

[92] Popoff, M.R., & Geny,B.(2009). Multifaceted role of Rho, Rac, Cdc42 and Ras in intercellular junctions, lessons from toxins. *Biochim Biophys Acta.* 1788:797-812.

[93] Gorvel, J.P., Chang, T.C., Boretto, J., Azuma, T., & Chavrier, P.(1988). Differential properties of D4/LyGDI versus RhoGDI: phosphorylation and rho GTPase selectivity. *FEBS Lett.* 422:269-273.

[94] Mège R.M., Gavard J., Lambert M.(2006). Regulation of cell-cell junctions by the cytoskeleton. *Curr Opin Cell Biol.* 18:541-548.

[95] Lin F., Chen S., Sepich D.S., Panizzi J.R., Clendenon S.G., Marrs J.A., Hamm H.E., Solnica-Krezel L.(2009). Galpha12/13 regulate epiboly by inhibiting E-cadherin 184:909-921.

[96] Yu, J., Vodyanik, M.A., Smuga-Otto, K., Antosiewicz-Bourget, J., Frane, J.L., Tian, S., Ni, J., Jonsdottir, G.A., Ruotti, V., Stewart, R.,

Slukvin, I.I., & Thomson J.A.(2007). Induced pluripotent stem cell lines *Science*. 318:1917-1920.

[97] Holm F., Ström S., Inzunza J., Baker D., Strömberg A.M., Rozell B., Feki A., Bergström R., Hovatta O.(2010). An effective serum- and xeno-free chemically defined freezing procedure for human embryonic and induced pluripotent stem cells. *Hum Reprod.* 25:1271-1279.

[98] Baharvand, H., Salekdeh, G.H., Taei, A., & Mollamohammadi, S.(2010). An efficient and easy-to-use cryopreservation protocol for human ES and iPS cells. *Nat Protoc.* 5:588-594.

[99] Claassen, D.A., Desler, M.M., Rizzino, A.(2010). ROCK innibition enhances the recovery and growth of cryopreserved human embryonic stem cells and human induced pluripotent stem cells. *Hum Reprod.* 25:1271-1279.

In: Induced Stem Cells
Editors: P. Sullivan and E. Mortensen

ISBN: 978-1-61324-613-9

Chapter II

Bone Tissue Engineering Approaches and Challenges Using Bioactive Ceramic Scaffolds

Manitha B. Nair
Department of Biomedical Engineering,
Georgia Institute of Technology, Atlanta, Georgia, USA

Abstract

Segmental bone defects resulting from trauma or pathological conditions represent formidable clinical challenges in orthopaedic surgery. Though current therapies include autografts and allografts or distraction osteogenesis, they are known for their inherent disadvantages like limited supply, increased morbidity, disease transmission potential and long term hospitalization respectively. In this context, tissue engineering becomes relevant for the treatment of large bone defects, where cells or growth factors are incorporated into a three-dimensional scaffold to mimic native tissue architecture and function in terms of osteoconduction, osteoinduction and osteointegration. Among the scaffolds, bioactive ceramics play an importance because of its similarity in chemical composition to bone. This review seeks to describe different tissue engineering approaches using bioactive ceramics towards bone regeneration in segmental bone defects. These include tissue-ingrowth (bioactive ceramics alone); cell transplantation (bioactive ceramics with mesenchymal stem cells) and signaling molecule (bioactive ceramics with growth factors).

1. Introduction

Bone has the remarkable capacity to heal without scar formation, but this regenerative process fails in patients with large bone lesions or impaired wound healing, requiring clinical intervention. Critical-sized segmental bone defects give rise to serious problems, where the defect does not heal spontaneously during the lifespan of the organism (Reichert JC et al., 2009). This leads to complications such as shortening of the structures, nerve and vascular lesions, cutaneous loss, delayed edema, and ultimately to the amputation of the involved member (DeCoster TA et al., 2004). Because of the absence of vascularisation and functional stimulation in these areas and together with the frequency of local infections, the treatment of these lesions are generally complex having a negative long-term impact on patient lives. Segmental bone defects can result either from acute trauma or chronic infection requiring bone resection or chronic non-unions due to osteoporosis or osteomyletis, osteogenesis imperfecta or osteosarcoma.

Current treatments for segmental defects include autografts or allografts or osteotomy followed by bone distraction (the Ilizarov technique). Autologous bone graft, harvested from iliac crest or fibula, has been the gold standard of bone replacement for many years because it provides osteogenic cells as well as essential osteoinductive and osteoconductive elements for healing (Morsi E 2002; Duffy GP et al., 2000). It has a success rate of 80% to 90% with no risks of immune rejection or disease transfer. However, the problems with autograft may at times offset the benefits. The supply is always limited to match the size of defects that occur in the long bones of lower limbs, e.g. femur and tibia (Abdollahi K et al., 1999). The harvesting of autograft requires an additional surgery and this adds a degree of morbidity and may involve massive blood loss, sepsis and pain, posing the patient for high risk (Betz RR, 2002). Another problem is late graft fracture, reported as high as 60% at 10 years, which is associated with a multitude of biologic processes such as osteoclastic resorption, increase in microfracture prevalence and decrease in bone mineral density (Wheeler DL and Enneking WF, 2005). Vail et al., (1996) reported

19% incidence of donor site morbidity in their series of 247 vascularised fibula grafts which includes symptoms of - more weakness, discomfort in the ankle and other sites in the leg and sensory abnormalities.

Allograft bone, usually from human cadaver, has been used extensively in the reconstruction of bone defects after tumor excision and is available in abundance. However, allograft demonstrates a lower osteogenic capacity so that the rate of incorporation of allograft is lower than with autograft (D'Agostino P et al., 2007). Additionally, it introduces the possibility of pathogen transfer from donor to host and although infrequent, infections ascribed to donor-host transmission following allografting procedures do occur. Hepatitis B (Tomford WW 1995) and Hepatitis C transmission (Conrad EU et al., 1995) have been reported with the transfer of allograft tissue.

The Ilizarov technique relies on the regeneration potential of bone, in which a corticotomy is followed by gradual movement of two cut ends of the bone (1 mm per day) using a circular external fixator. Besides the positive impact, there is a high chance of traction injury to nerves and other soft tissues. The pin track can become infected and a major neurovascular bundle may be punctured during pin placement. The docking site may need additional bone grafting for bony union. Thus this technique requires specialized training and equipment, long treatment durations and it is associated with frequent complications (Tomić S et al., 2007; Green SA et al., 1992).

Due to several problems associated with correct therapies and to improve countless lives of patients, demand for an ideal bone graft for the repair of segmental defects has become a dire necessity. The ideal bone substitutes are naturally those with biomechanical and biological properties most closely resembling those of normal bone and expected to be (a) Biocompatible (b) osteoconductive (c) osteointegrative (d) osteoinductive (e) osteogenic (Damien CJ et al., 1991). From the orthopaedic point of view, mechanical integrity, time-controlled degradation and simultaneous replacement by newly formed bone are the critical adequate factors in defining an ideal bone substitute. The mechanical integrity of the material can ensure the stability of limbs or sites with bone defects or even replace an internal or external fixation system during treatment (Kehr H et al., 1993). Time-controlled biodegradation of the material accommodates each step in biologic bone regeneration and remodeling to avoid a mechanically weakened stage during fracture or defect healing (Holmes RE 1979)

2. Bone Tissue Engineering

An important approach to develop an ideal bone graft is to allow natural tissues to regenerate at defect site by providing a structural support for the proliferation and differentiation of cells. Such an induction for regeneration can be achieved through "Tissue engineering", which is defined as "an interdisciplinary field of research that applies the principles of engineering and life sciences towards the development of biological substitutes that restore, maintain or improve tissue function" (Langer R and Vacanti JP, 1993). It utilizes a 3D porous biodegradable scaffold with cells and growth factors to fill the tissue void, to provide structural support and to regenerate tissue within the body upon transplantation. Thus the triad of tissue engineering consists of (a) 3D scaffold (b) cells and (c) growth factor, each of these can be used independently or in combination. Among them, the scaffold is the main component in determining the ultimate achievement of the tissue-engineered graft.

The scaffolds for bone tissue engineering include metals (Dabrowski B et al., 2010; Attias N et al., 2006), polymers like poly (lactic-co-glycolic acid) (PLGA) (*Bodde EW* et al., 2008; Isobe M et al., 1999); poly (LDL-lactide) (Gugala Z et al., 1999), polypropylene fumarate (Fisher JP et al; 2002) and ceramics. Each of these materials has its own advantages and disadvantages. For eg., metals like titanium cage alone (Shunsuke F et al., 2003) or titanium cage packed with a composite of cancellous allograft and demineralized bone matrix putty (Attias N et al., 2006) can achieve the torsional stiffness of lamellar bone in segmental defects. Nevertheless, these implants corrode in an *in vivo* environment, which can cause harmful effect on the surrounding tissues and organs (Høl PJ et al., 2008; *Singh R* and *Dahotre NB* 2007). Similarly, polymers failed to integrate with bone, leading to fibrous tissue formation and inflammation. Therefore the third group of scaffolds, i.e., bioactive ceramics like hydroxyapatite (HA) or tricalcium phosphate (TCP) is the most preferred biomaterial after autograft because of its similarity in chemical composition to bone apatite as described below.

3. Bioactive Ceramics

The bioactive ceramics like hydroxyapatite (HA) or tricalcium phosphate (TCP) (Wang M 2003), is the most preferred biomaterial after autograft because of its similarity in chemical composition to bone apatite. Biologically active hydroxyapatite carbonate layer (HCA) layer forms on the surface of these materials upon implantation, providing interfacial bond with bone (Wang M 2003). To describe further, when bioactive ceramics are placed in bone tissue, a gradual change on the ceramic surface occurs that leads to the dissolution of calcium and phosphate ions from HA. This process may either occur from surrounding environment (extracellular fluid) or may be mediated by osteoclasts. Dissolution generates increased concentration of calcium and inorganic phosphate in the space between the existing bone and the implant. The precipitation of HA into this space results in a HCA layer at the surface and promotes bonding of the implant with the bone without an intervening fibrous layer (Tachibana Y et al., 2003; Daculsi G et al., 1990).

The bioceramics that incorporate silica into their composition have also emphasized the importance of Si in the enhancement of bone growth (Carlisle EM 1980). These include materials with high Si levels like (a) Bioglass (b) apatite-wollastonite and (c) calcium phosphate based materials with trace levels of Si doping such as Si-HA and Si-TCP. Bioglass are melt-derived glasses having the base components of SiO_2, Na_2O, CaO and P_2O_5 in specific proportions. The first and most well studied composition termed Bioglass® 45S5 contains 45% SiO_2, 24.5% Na_2O, 24.4% CaO and 6% P_2O_5, all in weight percent, was introduced by Hench in 1970s (Hench LL et al., 1993). The second group of silicate glasses includes glass ceramics, which is prepared by melting and controlled crystallization method by Kokubo in 1982 (Hench LL et al., 1993). This glass ceramic was named apatite / wollastonite (A-W) after the names of crystalline phases. The bioactivity of glass ceramics is much higher than that of sintered HA (Wang M 2003). The third group is Si-substituted calcium phosphate ceramics, which includes Si-HA and Si-α-TCP. The synthesis of Si-HA and Si-α-TCP has focused on wet chemical methods where Si is introduced as a chemical carrier from tetraethyl or propyl ortho-silicate (TEOS or TPOS) to HA or TCP (Pietak AM et al., 2007). The phase composition of the materials are highly dependent on Ca / (P + Si) and Ca / P ratio of the system, the level of Si addition, the method of introducing Si to CaP and sintering conditions, most notably the sintering temperature.

Recently, a silica-based bioactive ceramic has been synhesized, namely HASi (Fig. 1). Instead of substituting silica in calcium phosphate ceramics, a layer of silica was coated by dipping sintered HA in silica sol prepared by the hydrolysis of TEOS in ethanol-water system for 1 min (sol gel method) and sintered at 1200°C for 2 h. The results have showed that the core of HASi was polycrystalline and has clear grain boundary characteristics, while the outer coated layer was porous, less crystalline and has no clear grain and grain boundary. The porous structure together with the absence of clear grain and grain boundary in the outer coated layer of HASi is expected due to Si rich liquid phase formation which has penetrated to a depth of about 1 mm (Nair MB et al., 2008; John et al., 2008).

On immersion in body fluids, silica based bioactive ceramics facilitate three general processes at the interface on the implant side: leaching, dissolution and precipitation. Leaching is characterized by a rapid exchange of sodium or potassium with H^+ and H_3O^+ ions in extracellular fluid, where the process is controlled by diffusion. Network dissolution occurs concurrently by breaking of Si-O-Si-O-Si bonds through the action of hydroxyl (OH) ions and form silicic acid [Si $(OH)_4$]. The hydrated silica (SiOH) undergoes rearrangements by polycondensation of neighboring silanols, resulting in a silica-rich gel layer. In the precipitation reaction, calcium and phosphate ions released from the material together with those from extracellular fluid form an amorphous calcium-phosphate-rich layer on the surface. It later crystallizes to form HCA structure by incorporating carbonate ions (OH^-, CO_3^{2-} or F^-) from the solution. Rapid growth of HCA agglomerates incorporates collagen fibrils that promote bonding with bone (Hench LL et al., 1993; Nordström EG et al., 2001).

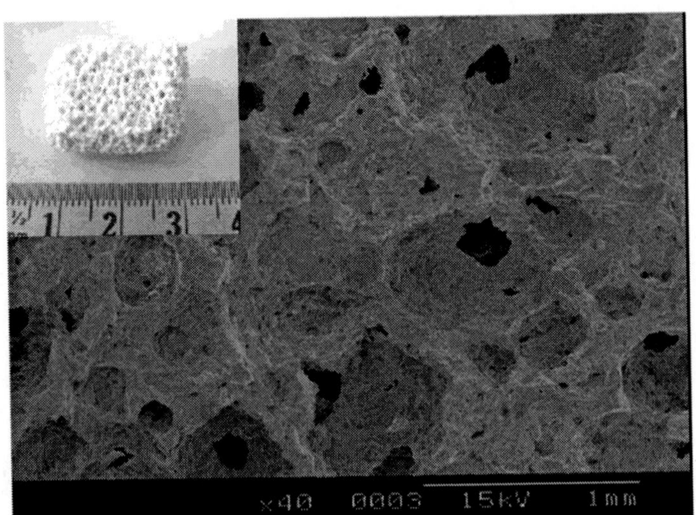

Figure 1. Scanning electron micrograph showing interconnected porous nature of HASi with pore size of 300 – 500 μm. The inset shows the gross view of the material (copied from Nair MB et al., Acta Biomater. 2008; 4(1): 173-81).

4. Tissue Engineering Approaches with Bioactive Ceramics

There are three tissue engineering approaches with bioactive ceramics, which are described below.

4.1. Tissue in-Growth

The bioceramics simply acts as a matrix to support the migration and proliferation of cell types from the host tissue to form a new tissue (osteoconduction only). Thus, healing is dependent upon the spreading and proliferation of indigenous or native cells on the scaffold. Studies have reported the use of materials like HA, TCP, HA-βTCP and coral for these applications.

Coralline HA and sintered TCP were evaluated to quantitate the bone ingrowth and biodegradability in the diaphysis of rabbit tibias (0.3 cm in diameter by 0.8 cm in length), the bone regeneration was noticed in two scaffolds, but HA did not show appreciable degradation until 24 weeks (Shimazaki K et al., 1985). In another study, a segmental defect (1 cm in rabbit ulna) was repaired with autogenous iliac crest bone, autogenous cortical bone (ulna), HA, HA-demineralized bone matrix composite graft, freeze-dried bone (allograft) and demineralized bone matrix in order to determine the appropriate substitute for autogenous grafts. The results showed that the demineralized bone matrix and HA-demineralized bone matrix composite graft is comparable in performance with autograft in mechanical strength and rate of union. On the contrary, freeze-dried bone and HA did not appear to be a suitable material for grafting segmental bone defects (Hopp SG et al., 1989). During the years from 1981 to 1986, HA was used in 45 patients, combined with autologous cancellous bone graft in 38 cases and used alone in seven cases to fill bone defects after removal of bone cysts and in trauma, for long fusions in patients with scoliosis, for non-union in lumbosacral area, for anterior vertebral fusions, in limb sparing operations for malignant bone tumours and in revised operations after failed joint endoprostheses. About 36 patients were reviewed up to sixty months after operation and the results were encouraging with no difference in progress compared with patients in whom simple autologous bone grafts had been used (Heise U et al., 1990). The cylinders of HA, bioactive glass and TCP showed bone-implant union when implanted in tibial segmental defects in sheep at 4 months (Gao TJ et al., 1995). When biocoral and TCP cylinders were implanted in osteotomized sheep tibial defects (1.6 cm in length), better osteointegration and biomechanical performance was observed in biocoral cylinders and seemed to be superior to TCP after 16 weeks (Gao TJ et al., 1997). Porous ceramic cylinders consisting of HA (65%) and β-TCP (35%) showed a radiographic union at the interface between host bone and implants when implanted in the femora (2.1 cm) of adult female dogs. A small amount of trabecular bone formed at the cut ends of the cortex of host bone, but the mid region of defect was filled with fibrous tissue (Bruder SP et al., 1998). Extensive integration of HA with host bone was detected when implanted in tibial diaphyseal defect (3.5 cm) of adult sheep (Marcacci M et al., 1999). The use of coral as a scaffold material was ineffective in the healing of goat femur segmental defect (2.5 cm) (Zhu et al., 2006). When porous interconnected HA and HA / TCP (60 / 40) ceramics were used in segmental bone defects in rabbits, the densities at the bone-ceramic interface decreased gradually with time indicating its limited application in the treatment of segmental bone defects (Balçik C et al., 2007). When β-TCP was used for 3 cm mandibular segmental defect, minimal bone formation with almost fibrous connection was observed (Yuan et al., 2007).

4.1.1. Challenges

Some of these studies have shown promising results, while others have showed the disadvantages of these materials for segmental defects. In most studies, the main problem encountered was related to the degradation nature of HA or TCP. HA is resistant to resorption *in vivo*, which occurs at a rate of 1 - 2% per year, so that full repair or function or remodeling of bone could be limited because of long term foreign sequestration in the body (Constantino PD and Friedman CD, 1994). On the other hand, TCP was found to resorb within days to weeks in vitro and in vivo and the bone volume produced will always be less than the volume of TCP resorbed (Holinger JO et al., 1996). Additionally, a few studies have shown fibrous tissue deposition in the mid portion of the defects (Bruder et al., 1998; Zhu et al., 2006), where the migration and proliferation rate of native cells may not have matched with the degradation rate of scaffold, resulting in fibrous union.

4.2. Cell Transplantation

In the second approach of Tissue engineering, the cells isolated from the patient are cultured on the scaffold and is transplanted into the defect site. The outcome in these studies is better because the cells could efficiently proliferate and produce their own extracellular matrix (ECM) on the scaffold and thereby decrease the time needed for the biosynthetic activity from indigenous osteoprogenitors. These cells can also secrete inductive factors that recruit indigenous mesenchymal stem cells (MSCs) into osteogenic lineage and produce mature bone matrix quickly. Thus the combined contribution from cells on the scaffolds and host-derived MSCs together with biomolecules can advance osteogenesis at the defect site.

4.2.1. Mesenchymal Stem Cells

In bone tissue engineering, there has been special interest in stem cells located in the bone marrow known as mesenchymal stem cells. MSCs have shown extensive capacity for expansion *in vitro*, so these cells have been considered as candidates for cell therapy. These cells can differentiate into multiple cell lineages including bone, cartilage, muscle, bone marrow stroma, tendon / ligament, fat, dermis, and other connective tissues (Caplan AI 1990; Caplan AI 1991; Caplan AI 2005). The multipotency of MSCs has been further exemplified by the observation that after the transplantation of these cells into a host animal, an ectopic ossicle consisting of osteoblastic, adipogenic and chondrogenic tissue phenotypes has been developed (Mauney JR et al., 2005). Also MSCs themselves, secrete a broad spectrum of bioactive macromolecules that are both immunoregulatory and serve to structure a regenerative microenvironment in the arena of tissue injury.

MSCs were first described in the 1970s by Friedenstein et al., who discovered that the cells adhered to tissue culture plates, resembled fibroblasts *in vitro*, and formed colonies (Friedenstein AJ et al 1970). Later Caplan gave these cells the name they have today, mesenchymal stem cells (Caplan AI 1991). MSCs have been found in several tissue locations, including bone marrow (Malgieri A et al., 2010), fat (Kroeze RJ et al., 2011), umbilical cord blood (Seong JM et al., 2010), periosteum (Diaz-Flores et al., 1992; Nakahara et al., 1991), peritrabecular connective tissue (Ishida H et al., 1993) and even peripheral blood (Kuznetsov SA et al 2001). The differentiation characteristics, the purity, and the yields are quite different for all of the stem cell preparations from different tissues. Therefore, the defining characteristics of MSCs are inconsistent among investigators. To address this problem, the

Mesenchymal and Tissue Stem Cell Committee of the International Society for Cellular Therapy (ISCT) proposes a set of standards to define human MSC for both laboratory-based scientific investigations and for pre-clinical studies (Horwitz E et al., 2005). First, MSC must be plastic-adherent when maintained in standard culture conditions using tissue culture flasks. Second, ≥ 95% of the MSC population must express CD105, CD73 and CD90, as measured by flow cytometry. Additionally, these cells must lack expression (≤2% positive) of CD45, CD34, CD14 or CD11b, CD79a or CD19 and HLA class II. Third, the cells must be able to differentiate to osteoblasts, adipocytes and chondroblasts under standard *in vitro* differentiating conditions (Dominici M et al., 2006). However, these characteristics were not defined cells from other species.

Through the addition of osteogenic supplements including dexamethasone, ascorbic acid and β-glycerophosphate, purified culture-expanded MSCs can be differentiated into osteogenic lineage *in vitro*, as envisaged by the production of collagen-rich matrix, increased expression of non-collagenous proteins like ALP, osteocalcin and finally by the formation of mineralized matrix (Kern S et al., 2006). Ascorbic acid is required for the synthesis of collagen and for osteogenesis *in vitro* (Maehata Y et al., 2006). It also regulates ALP activity and protein synthesis in osteoblast cultures (Son E et al., 2007). The organic phosphate, β glycerophosphate, has often been used *in vitro* to provide a potential source of phosphate ions for mineralization (zur Nieden NI et al., 2003). Dexamethasone, the key factor in producing bone-like nodules, is a synthetic glucocorticoid. One signal transduction pathway that has been associated with dexamethasone is the signaling of Wnt, which is a secreted glycoprotein that exerts concentration-dependent effect on cell fate (de Boer J et al., 2004). Wnt activates β- catenin resulting in its nuclear translocation that leads to an increased expression of Runx2 and ALP (Hamidouche Z et al., 2008). Studies have demonstrated that the osteogenic differentiation potential of MSCs decreases after serial passaging (Sugiura F et al., 2004; Ter Brugge PJ et al., 2002). Serial passaging has been found to alter surface marker expression, which reflects a marked change in the response of MSCs to chemical stimuli that promote osteogenesis (Wall ME et al., 2007).

4.2.2. Mesenchymal Stem Cells for Cell Transplantation

The first cell-based attempt for bone tissue engineering was focused on fresh autologous or syngenic bone marrow, a source of osteogenic cells. The addition of autologous bone marrow to HA ceramics did improve healing of a segmental defect (3 cm) in the midshaft of sheep tibia (Wippermann B et al., 1999). The combination of resorbable calcium phosphate ceramics with autologous bone marrow does not provide an alternative for autologous bone grafting in a 3 cm tibial segmental defect (Blokhuis TJ et al., 2000). When a 3 cm segmental defect in the tibia of sheep model was repaired with autologous bone marrow and HA, bony bridging in the defect was enhanced than with HA alone group (den Boer FC et al., 2003).

In most of the studies, the addition of bone marrow did not improve bone healing because of the insufficient number of osteoprogenitors in bone marrow, especially as age increases. When grouped by decade, a dramatic decrease in MSCs per nucleated marrow cell could be observed with a 10-fold decrease from birth to teens and another 10-fold decrease from teens to the elderly (In adults, it is present at concentrations of less than 1 in 100, 000 – 500, 000 nucleated cells in bone marrow aspirates) (Caplan AI, 2007).

Therefore, the current state of art within bone tissue engineering consists of the combination of culture-expanded MSCs with 3D porous biomaterials. In 1997, Kadyala et al., showed that MSCs in combination with porous ceramic scaffolds could repair segmental defects (0.8 cm) in the femora of rats in 8 weeks. Human MSCs loaded ceramics were significantly stronger and regenerated bone in segmental defect in the femur of adult athymic rats at 12 weeks (Bruder SP et al., 1998b). Autologous MSCs cultured onto porous ceramic cylinders consisting of HA (65%) and β-TCP (35%) regenerated lamellar bone throughout the defect (2.1 cm) in canine model at 16 weeks (Bruder SP et al., 1998a). The use of autologous MSCs in conjunction with HA resulted in faster bone repair compared to HA alone when implanted in tibia of sheep model (Kon E et al., 2000). The bone defect (2.1 cm) in the femoral diaphysis of adult dogs was repaired with allogeneic MSCs loaded onto a hollow ceramic cylinder consisting of HA-TCP. Histologically by eight weeks, a callus spanned the length of the defect and at sixteen weeks, new bone had formed throughout the implant (Arinzeh TL et al., 2003). Engineering bones with porous TCP and autologous MSCs in sheep metatarsus were capable of repairing segmental defect (2.5 cm) almost completely at 24 weeks in the creep substitution way without progression through a cartilaginous intermediate (Li Z et al., 2005). Highly porous HA scaffolds loaded with *in vitro* expanded MSCs depicted new bone from week 8 and was arrested at week 24 (Komlev VS et al., 2006) in immunodeficient mice. Autogenous BMSCs with β-TCP ensured bone formation and vascularisation throughout the defects (3 cm) in the mandibles of the dog (He Y et al., 2007).

Although the implantation of MSC-seeded biomaterials has shown significant increase in skeletal repair, additional *in vitro* culture methods have been developed that promote osteogenic differentiation of MSCs *in vitro* in lieu of *in vivo* incorporation. These cell-loaded ceramics have succeeded in creating bone formation in animal models (Liu G et al., 2008; Nair et al., 2009c; Nair et al., 2009d).

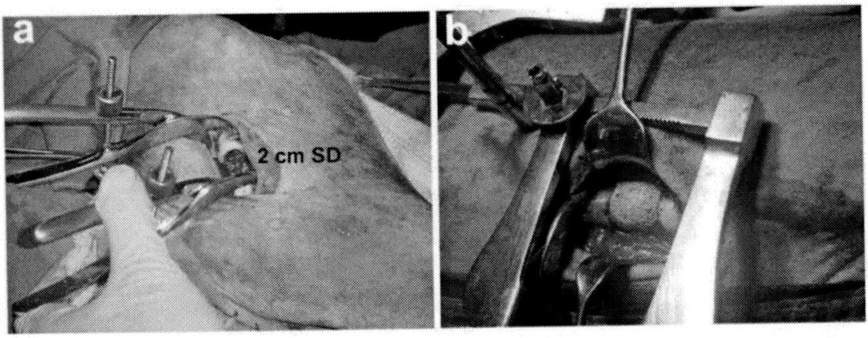

Figure 2. The photographs of surgical procedure (a) segmental defect (2 cm) created in the femur of goat model (b) HASi implanted at the defect site (copied from Nair MB et al., Acta Biomater. 2009; 5(5):1742-55).

The possibility of engineering bone in a goat model has also been tested using osteogenic induced bone marrow-derived MSCs and HASi. The cells were cultured on the bioactive ceramic for 1 week before the transplantation. In the surgical procedure, a 2 cm segmental defect was created in the femur of the goat model and the defect was treated with tissue-engineered HASi (HASi+C) and HASi alone (Fig. 2). The materials were stabilized with titanium intramedullay nails and screws. In bare HASi groups, lamellar pattern of bone formation was seen only in the peripheral region, while the mid region was filled with woven bone at 4 months. The mid region was later organized into lamellar pattern at 6 months and a complete bone remodeling at 12 months. Interestingly, in HASi+C groups, a mature lamellar pattern of newly formed bone was observed throughout the defect at 4 months. Thus, whatever the qualities attained in the tissue-engineered groups at 2 months was achievable only at 4 months in bare HASi groups (Fig. 3). This may be due to the combined osteoinductive and osteoconductive effect of HASi+C groups (Nair et al., 2009d; Nair MB et al., 2010)

It was observed that the culture of cells on HASi could not only enhance bone regeneration, but also mediate material degradation (HASi degraded faster in HASi+C groups than HASi alone groups – Fig. 4), which is one of the main problems encountered in the category of tissue-ingrowth. It is hypothesized that osteogenic induced MSCs cultured on HASi create an ECM that can favor the successive migration of osteoclasts. Among many ECM proteins, osteopontin has an important role in promoting the adhesion of osteoclasts to the scaffold surface through their arginine-glycine-aspartic acid sequence (Mastrogiacomo M et al., 2006). *In vitro* studies have shown that the expression of osteopontin was significantly enhanced on HASi than HA (Nair MB et al., 2009b). Thus the combined effects of the characteristics of the material (porosity and silica content) and the ability of cells on HASi to attract osteoclasts have improved cell-mediated resorption in HASi+C groups.

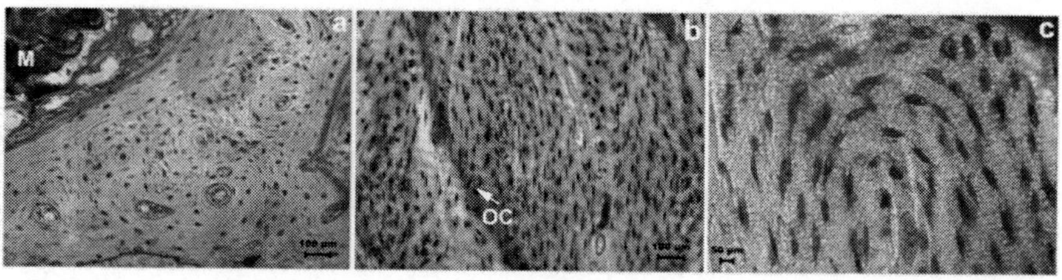

Figure 3. Histological examination of the treated defect demonstrated union with new bone formation - Stevenel's blue and Van Gieson's picro fuchsin staining (a) HASi (b) HASi+C (c) The magnified view (40x) of figure 3b (OC- osteocyte, M – Material) (copied from Nair MB et al., J Biomed Mater Res A. 2009; 91(3):855-65).

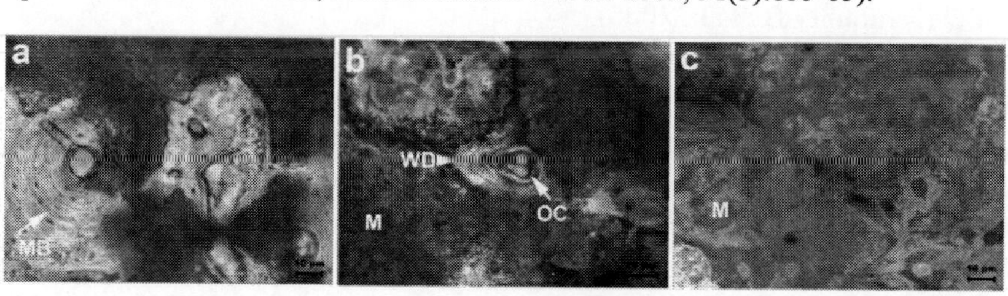

Figure 4. Histology showing bone resorption by osteoclasts and bone apposition on the remnants of the material in HASi+C group - Stevenel's blue and Van Gieson's picro fuchsin staining (a) Haversian systems in contact with material (b) Bone resorption process in par with new bone formation on the material (50x) (c) Osteoclast-mediated resorption (100x). WB-woven bone; MB – mature bone; M-material; OC-osteoclast (copied from Nair MB et al., Acta Biomater. 2009; 5(5):1742-55).

4.2.3. Challenges

The formation of bone is directly related to the number of cells seeded on the scaffold (Fleming JE Jr et al., 2000). Bruder et al., (1998c) suggested that excessively high concentrations of bone marrow-derived MSCs are disadvantageous in their adherence to scaffold. However, none of the reports have mentioned the exact number of cells grown on 3D porous ceramics for transplantation. This is because of the technical difficulty to count the entire number of cells on the inner and outer side of the 3D scaffold.

Apart from cell number, the *in vitro* culture period of tissue-engineered constructs also influences their ability to regenerate bone when implanted in segmental defects. One study reported that sintered titanium fiber meshes seeded with cells that have been cultured in osteogenic media for 4 days revealed the highest bone formation when implanted in cranial defect of Fisher rats and lowest bone formation was obtained when it was cultured for 16 days in vitro (Castano-Izquierdo H et al., 2007). Based on these findings, a seven day *in vitro* culture period was done prior to transplantation. More focus in this area is necessary since the culture period affects the ECM deposition that influences the rate of bone formation.

An additional problem encountered is the levels of heterogeneity within the MSC cultures and their differentiation *in vitro*. For eg. one study has shown the presence of two kinds of cell populations, i. e, spindle-shaped and flat shaped MSCs. The number of flat cells increased over time in all cultures and has shown to lose differentiation potential. It is not clear if these spindle-shaped cells represent recently divided flat MSC that will shortly reacquire the flat phenotype, or if they are a subpopulation that can be re-derived from flat MSC (Neuhuber B et al., 2008).

In recent years, studies of human MSCs age-related factors have at times yielded differing results. Although associations between increased donor age and decreased osteoprogenitor numbers have been reported (Nishida S et al., 1999; Stenderup K et al., 2003), the impact of age on osteogenic differentiation is controversial. Some reports indicate that osteogenic potential decreases with age (Martinez ME et al., 1999; D'Ippolito G et al., 1999], whereas others state that MSCs retain the potential to differentiate (Leskela HV et al., 2003; Fickert S et al., 2010]. Another major finding in this area is the number of MSCs harvested per bone marrow aspirate (Muschler GF et al., 2001) and its differentiation towards osteogenic lineage potential (Fickert S et al., 2010) is dependent on gender. This capability was relatively low in women when compared to men.

Another study emphasized the importance of aspiration volume of human bone marrow. For that, a study was conducted with aspiration volumes of two and four milliliters. The results showed that an increase in the aspiration volume from one to four milliliters caused a decrease of approximately 50 per cent in the final concentration of alkaline phosphatase positive colony-forming units in an average sample. This is because a larger volume decreases the concentration of osteoblast progenitor cells because of dilution of the bone-marrow sample with peripheral blood (Muschler GF et al., 1997).

Because of all these issues, many studies have shown variations in the results in this application.

In this context, questions of high clinical relevance remain unanswered: 1) For a given transplantation therapy, what defines the target subpopulation of MSC, 2) how should this subpopulation be culture-expanded on 3D scaffolds, and 3) how should the culture period be optimized to get a standard cell number and ECM deposition before and after transplantation?

4.3. Signaling Molecules

In the third approach of Tissue engineering, the growth factors are delivered to the defect site either directly or indirectly by encapsulation in the biomaterial. Studies related to bioceramics are limited in this application. When bFGF gene modified MSCs seeded on porous β-TCP ceramics and grafted into 1.5 cm segmental bone defect in the radius of New Zealand white rabbits, bone healing was accelerated through capillary regeneration (Guo X et al., 2006). The release of BMP-2 from the encapsulated PLGA / HA composite scaffolds increased the bioactivity of the material leading to improved new bone formation in segmental defects in vivo (Fu YC et al., 2008). The cost of almost all genetically engineered growth factors is prohibitively high, which limits its use for large defects where large amount of growth factors are needed. Thus researchers have looked for some other source that can deliver growth factors. For eg., platelet-rich plasma (PRP) and fibrin glue (FG).

4.3.1. Platelet-Rich Plasma

Platelet-rich plasma is a proven source of many growth factors like platelet-derived growth factor (PDGF), transforming growth factor-beta (TGF-β), vascular endothelial growth factor (VEGF) and insulin-like growth factor (IGF-I) (Anitua E et al., 2007). Some studies have shown promising results related to PRP. For eg. the bilateral implantation of polycaprolactone-TCP composite with PRP into 0.8 cm rat femoral defects accelerated early vascular ingrowth and improved longer-term functional integration when compared to a group without PRP after 3 weeks (Rai B et al., 2007). On the other hand, some reports haven shown that PRP did not influence bone healing (Mooren RE et al., 2007; Choi BH et al., 2004).

The therapeutic osteogenic effect of local platelet administration depends on the concentration of platelets and growth factors, which is dependent on the method of the preparation of PRP, (Weibrich G et al., 2003). A platelet count of 1000 x 10^6 / mL measured in a volume of 5 mL plasma is considered as the "therapeutic dose" of PRP (van den Dolder J et al., 2006 and Landesberg R et al., 2000). Platelet concentration of less than 1000 x 10^6 / mL were not reliable to enhance wound healing, whereas higher concentrations also did not show any further enhancement of wound healing (Marx RE et al., 2001). Additionally, the life span of a platelet and the period of direct influence of its growth factors are less than 5 days in an *in vivo* situation (Marx RE et al., 1998), which should be taken into consideration.

It is reported that the growth factors are released from platelets when they are activated with triggering agents like bovine thrombin or calcium chloride. Therefore, PRP is applied as gel by combining with these triggering factors. Nevertheless, recently, some studies have reported the negative effect of PRP gel when compared to PRP liquid. An explanation projected is that PRP gel has a viscous jelly-like consistency, which can result in additional pressure on the drill walls of already tightly fitted implant. This might cause an additional trauma during its installation and as a result, the healing process at bone-implant interface might become disturbed (Nikolidakis D et al., 2006). Significantly more interfacial bone-to-implant contact was attained while using PRP in liquid form than in the form of gels (Nikolidakis D et al., 2006). Additionally, the use of bovine thrombin has been reported to be associated with the development of antibodies to factor V and XI, which can result in the risk of life threatening coagulopathies (Landesberg R et al., 1998).

Based on these reports, we have focused on the delivery of PRP liquid into the defect site in the absence of triggering factors with calcium chloride and thrombin. We have isolated PRP from the blood of goat and humans by centrifuging at 2500 rpm for 5 min. The platelet count of goat PRP was about 600 x 10^6 platelets / mL whereas the platelet counts of human PRP was about 400 x 10^6 platelets / mL. Even though the isolation procedure adopted was same for both species, it resulted in two different platelet counts. Thus, this factor is of concern when extrapolating the results of animals into humans. As a preliminary step, we have coated PRP on HA and HASi by immersing these materials in PRP for 1h with agitation. The results showed that platelets adhered and get activated on these materials without the use of triggering agents (Nair et al., 2009). The activation was significantly enhanced on HASi than HA where the chemical composition, particularly silica may have played an important role (Nemmar A et al., 2005).

For *in vivo* study, the PRP was delivered as a liquid into a 2 cm segmental defect in the femur of goat model (9 mL of PRP having a count of 600 x10^6 / mL platelets was added so that a therapeutic dose of 5400 x 10^6 / 9 mL can be expected at the defect site). Quantitatively, there was no significant difference between HASi+C (with osteogenic induced MSCs only) and HASi+CP (with osteogenic induced MSCs + PRP) groups in terms of bone regeneration and material degradation. Nevertheless, HASi+CP groups showed a better response qualitatively where the lamellar bone was more organized (Nair et al., 2009c). In general, it is understood that that PRP does not have any strong osteogenic effect so that filling a defect with PRP alone will not allow osteogenesis to occur in larger defects. Instead, PRP has an osteopromotive effect and can enhance bone regeneration in the presence of osteogenic precursor cells by encouraging their proliferation and differentiation (Schlegel KA et al., 2004). Additionally, MSCs associated with PRP are potent angiogenic inducers proven to release VEGF leading to faster bone regeneration and remodeling (Lucarelli E et al., 2005; Yamada Y et al., 2004). Kitoh et al., (2007 and 2004) observed that transplantation of bone marrow cells and PRP shortened treatment period and reduced associated complications by accelerating new bone formation in distraction osteogenesis

4.3.2. Fibrin Glue

Another example is fibrin glue, which is a biopolymer matrix commonly used for surgical homeostasis and tissue sealing and is known to be critical in the normal wound healing process (Albala DM 2003; Jackson MR 2001). Fibrin glue contains smaller amounts of many growth factors like TGF-β, bFGF, epidermal growth factor (EGF) and VEGF (Ho W et al., 2006). *In vitro* studies indicate that FG can support the growth, migration and differentiation of several cell types: MSCs (Bensaïd W et al., 2003), endothelial cells (Sporn LA et al., 1995) and fibroblast cells (Meana A et al., 1998). Different biomaterials such as coral, bone-derived materials, bioactive glass ceramics and synthetic calcium phosphate have been mixed with FG, resulting in a significant positive effect on osteointegration and bone colonization (Le Guéhennec L et al., 2004). The osteoinductive potential of fibrin has been implicated based on a study with FG and calcium phosphate calcium silicate system, where new bone formation was observed at an extraskeletal site (muscle) in mice at day 15 (Abiraman et al., 2002). Similar results were obtained by Yamada et al., (2003) with the association of β-TCP-FG-MSC at 8 weeks in heterotopic sites in rats.

HA and HASi has been coated also with fibrin glue. *In vitro* studies have proved that FG coated HA and HASi can enhance cell performance (proliferation and osteogenic differentiation) when compared to PRP coated and uncoated materials (FG coated > PRP coated > uncoated), with preference towards HASi than HA (Fig. 5). The cell cycle analysis (PI staining by flow cytometry) has shown that percentage of cells in apoptotic phase was lower on coated materials than uncoated materials (Nair MB et al., 2009a). FG contains arginine-glycine-asparagine (RGD) motifs, which bind to cell receptors (predominately integrins) very firmly and sustain cellular viability (Sierra DH 1993).

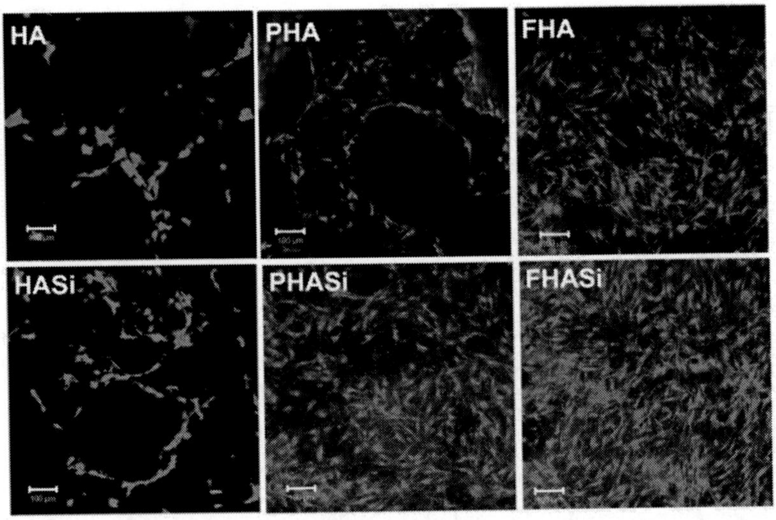

Figure 5. Confocal laser scanning micrograph showing the viability (calcein staining - green) of osteogenic-induced gBMSCs cultured on uncoated, PRP and FG coated HA and HASi over 28 days. (copied from Nair MB et al., Tissue Eng Part A. 2009; 15(7):1619-31.

For *in vivo* studies, some of the features of PRP are attractive in their use when compared to FG. These include (a) they can be easily obtained from patient's blood after a simple centrifugation step (b) PRP contains high concentration of platelets and a native concentration of fibrinogen. Thus, the effect of FG also will be attained in the presence of indigenous thrombin when PRP is delivered to the defect site (Yamada Y et al., 2004) (c) PRP preparation is cheap while the cost of commercially available FG like Tisseel is exorbitant for its price (Alving B et al., 1999).

4.3.3. Challenges

There are controversies in the literature regarding the potential benefits of PRP. In effect, some authors have reported improvements in tissue healing and bone formation using PRP and others failed to observe such positive effect. Such discrepancies are probably related to the lack of suitable standardization and definition of the different PRP preparations; different protocols and biological / surgical techniques used in the elaboration and administration of the PRP (Anitua E et al., 2006). Thus procedures need to be standardized and well-designed studies and clinical trials are needed to evaluate the potential therapeutic impact of PRP in medicine and surgery and to avoid controversial results.

The use of fibrin glue in the operating room, consists of cryoprecipitate (usually allogeneic from the blood bank) mixed with an equal volume of bovine thrombin (Alving BM et al., 1995). Preparations from some manufacturers contain sufficient bovine factor V to induce antibodies in the recipient that then cross react with the recipient's factor V and result in a bleeding diathesis 7 to 10 days after surgery (Christie RJ et al., 1997). To overcome this problem, highly purified, virally inactivated fibrin sealant is now commercially available in the United States (Tisseel; manufactured by Immuno AG). However, the cost is high (about $300) for a final preparation that has a total volume of 4 mL. Therefore, alternatives to improve the usage of FG have to be investigated.

Conclusion

Segmental bone defects caused by tumor resections, trauma, and skeletal abnormalities such as osteomyelitis remain a major problem in orthopedics because of the lack of predictability in attaining functional bone after the treatment. The current treatments like autograft, allograft or distraction osteogenesis are associated with several limitations. Therefore, researchers are focusing on a new concept called "Tissue engineering" in which 3D porous biodegradable scaffolds are incorporated with cells or growth factors to regenerate tissue within the body. Over the years, a number of scaffolds have emerged and among these, bioactive ceramics are most preferred because of its similarity in chemical composition to bone apatite. In this review, three tissue-engineering approaches using bioactive ceramics have been summarized (a) Tissue-in growth – scaffold simply acts as a matrix to support the migration and proliferation of indigenous cell types to form a new tissue (b) Cell transplantation - The cells isolated from the patient are cultured on the scaffold *in vitro* and transplanted into the defect site so that the cells could efficiently proliferate and produce their own extracellular matrix (ECM) on the scaffold (c) signaling molecules - the recombinant growth factors or PRP / FG delivered to the defect site either directly or after encapsulation in the biomaterial. Although significant results have been achieved with the three approaches, there are many challenges that are to be addressed before any of the described strategies become a clinical reality in future.

Acknowledgments

The authors acknowledge The Director, SCTIMST for the facilities provided to carry out the work; Dr. H. K. Varma for bioceramics; Dr. K.V.Menon and Dr. Sachin J Shenoy for the goat surgical procedures; DRDO for financial assistance; and CSIR for the fellowship to Dr. M.B.N.

References

Abdollahi K, Kumar PJ, Shepherd L, Patzakis MJ. Estimation of defect volume in segmental defects of the tibia and femur. *J Trauma*. 1999; 46(3): 413-6.

Abiraman S, Varma HK, Umashankar PR, John A. Fibrin glue as an osteoinductive protein in a mouse model. *Biomaterials* 2002; 23(14): 3023-31.

Albala DM. Fibrin sealants in clinical practice. *Cardiovasc Surg*. 2003; 11 Suppl 1: 5-11.

Alving BM, Weinstein MJ, Finlayson JS, Menitove JE, Fratantoni JC. Fibrin sealant: summary of a conference on characteristics and clinical uses. *Transfusion*. 1995; 35(9):783-90.

Anitua E, Sánchez M, Nurden AT, Nurden P, Orive G, Andía I. New insights into and novel applications for platelet-rich fibrin therapies. *Trends Biotechnol*. 2006; 24(5): 227-34.

Anitua E, Sánchez M, Nurden AT, Nurden P, Orive G, Andía I. New insights into and novel applications for platelet-rich fibrin therapies.*Trends Biotechnol*. 2006; 24(5):227-34.

Arinzeh TL, Peter SJ, Archambault MP, van den Bos C, Gordon S, Kraus K, Smith A, Kadiyala S. Allogeneic mesenchymal stem cells regenerate bone in a critical-sized canine segmental defect. *J Bone Joint Surg Am*. 2003; 85-A(10): 1927-35.

Attias N, Lindsey RW. Case reports: management of large segmental tibial defects using a cylindrical mesh cage. *Clin Orthop Relat Res*. 2006; 450: 259- 66.

Balçik C, Tokdemir T, Senköylü A, Koç N, Timuçin M, Akin S, Korkusuz P, Korkusuz F. Early weight bearing of porous HA/TCP (60/40) ceramics in vivo: a longitudinal study in a segmental bone defect model of rabbit. *Acta Biomater*. 2007; 3(6): 985-96.

Bensaïd W, Triffitt JT, Blanchat C, Oudina K, Sedel L, Petite H. A biodegradable fibrin scaffold for mesenchymal stem cell transplantation. *Biomaterials* 2003; 24(14): 2497-502.

Betz RR. Limitations of autograft and allograft: new synthetic solutions.*Orthopedics*. 2002;25(5 Suppl):s561-70.

Blokhuis TJ, Wippermann BW, den Boer FC, van Lingen A, Patka P, Bakker FC, Haarman HJ. Resorbable calcium phosphate particles as a carrier material for bone marrow in an ovine segmental defect. *J Biomed Mater Res*. 2000; 51(3): 369-75.

Bodde EW, Spauwen PH, Mikos AG, Jansen JA. Closing capacity of segmental radius defects in rabbits.*J Biomed Mater Res A*. 2008; 85(1):206-17.

Bruder SP, Kraus KH, Goldberg VM, Kadiyala S. The effect of implants loaded with autologous mesenchymal stem cells on the healing of canine segmental bone defects. *Bone Joint Surg Am*. 1998a; 80(7): 985-96.

Bruder SP, Kurth AA, Shea M, Hayes WC, Jaiswal N, Kadiyala S. Bone regeneration by implantation of purified, culture-expanded human mesenchymal stem cells. *J Orthop Res*. 1998b; 16(2): 155-62.

Bruder SP, Kurth AA, Shea M, Hayes WC, Jaiswal N, Kadiyala S. Bone regeneration by implantation of purified, culture-expanded human mesenchymal stem cells. *J Orthop Res*. 1998c; 16(2):155-62.

Caplan AI. Adult mesenchymal stem cells for tissue engineering versus regenerative medicine.*J Cell Physiol*. 2007; 213(2):341-7.

Caplan AI. Cell delivery and tissue regeneration. *Journal of Controlled Release* 1990; 11: 157-165.

Caplan AI. Mesenchymal stem cells. *J Orthop Res* 1991; 9: 641–650.

Caplan AI. Review: Mesenchymal stem cells: Cell-based reconstructive therapy in orthopedics. *Tissue Eng* 2005; 11: 1198–1211.

Carlisle EM. Biochemical and morphological changes associated with long bone abnormalities in silicon deficiency. *J Nutr.* 1980; 110(5):1046-56.

Castano-Izquierdo H, Alvarez-Barreto J, van den Dolder J, Jansen JA, Mikos AG, Sikavitsas VI. Pre-culture period of mesenchymal stem cells in osteogenic media influences their in vivo bone forming potential. *J Biomed Mater Res.* A 2007; 82(1): 129-38.

Choi BH, Im CJ, Huh JY, Suh JJ, Lee SH. Effect of platelet-rich plasma on bone regeneration in autogenous bone graft. *Int J Oral Maxillofac Surg.* 2004; 33(1): 56-9.

Christie RJ, Carrington L, Alving B. Postoperative bleeding induced by topical bovine thrombin: report of two cases.*Surgery.* 1997;121(6):708-10.

Conrad EU, Gretch DR, Obermeyer KR, et al. Transmission of the hepatitis-C virus by tissue transplantation. *J Bone Joint Surg Am.* 1995; 77(2):214-24.

Constantino PD, Friedman CD. Synthetic bone graft substitutes. *Otolaryngol Clin North Am* 1994; 27: 1037-73.

Dabrowski B, Swieszkowski W, Godlinski D, Kurzydlowski KJ. Highly porous titanium scaffolds for orthopaedic applications.*J Biomed Mater Res B Appl Biomater.* 2010;95(1):53-61.

Daculsi G, LeGeros RZ, Deudon C. Scanning and transmission electron microscopy, and electron probe analysis of the interface between implants and host bone. Osseo-coalescence versus osseo-integration. *Scanning Microsc.* 1990; 4(2): 309-14.

D'Agostino P, Stassen P, Delloye C. Post-traumatic bone loss of the femur treated with segmental bone allograft and bone morphogenetic protein: a case report. *Acta Orthop Belg.* 2007; 73(3): 396-9.

Damien CJ, Parsons JR. Bone graft and bone graft substitutes: a review of current technology and applications *J Appl Biomater.* 1991; 2(3): 187-208.

De Boer J, Wang HJ, Van Blitterswijk C. Effects of Wnt signaling on proliferation and differentiation of human mesenchymal stem cells. *Tissue Eng.* 2004; 10(3-4): 393-401.

DeCoster TA, Gehlert RJ, Mikola EA, Pirela-Cruz MA. Management of posttraumatic segmental bone defects. *J Am Acad Orthop Surg.* 2004: 12(1): 28-38.

den Boer FC, Wippermann BW, Blokhuis TJ, Patka P, Bakker FC, Haarman HJ. Healing of segmental bone defects with granular porous hydroxyapatite augmented with recombinant human osteogenic protein-1 or autologous bone marrow. *J Orthop Res.* 2003; 21(3): 521-8.

Diaz-Flores, L.; Gutierrez, R.; Lopez-Alonso, A.; Gonzalez, R.; and Varela, H.: Pericytes as a supplementary source of osteoblasts in periosteal osteogenesis. *Clin. Orthop.,* 275:280-286,1992.

D'Ippolito G, Schiller PC, Ricordi C, Roos BA, Howard GA.. Age-related osteogenic potential of mesenchymal stromal stem cells from human vertebral bone marrow. *J Bone Miner Res* 1999; 14:1115–1122.

Dominici M, Le Blanc K, Mueller I, Slaper-Cortenbach I, Marini F, Krause D, Deans R, Keating A, Prockop Dj, Horwitz E. Minimal criteria for defining multipotent mesenchymal stromal cells. The International Society for Cellular Therapy position statement. *Cytotherapy*. 2006; 8(4):315-7.

Duffy GP, Wood MB, Rock MG, Sim FH. Vascularized free fibular transfer combined with autografting for the management of fracture nonunions associated with radiation therapy. *J Bone Joint Surg Am*. 2000; 82(4): 544-54.

Fickert S, Schröter-Bobsin U, Groß AF, Hempel U, Wojciechowski C, Rentsch C, Corbeil D, Günther KP.Human mesenchymal stem cell proliferation and osteogenic differentiation during long-term ex vivo cultivation is not age dependent. *J Bone Miner Metab*. 2010.

Fisher JP, Vehof JW, Dean D, van der Waerden JP, Holland TA, Mikos AG, Jansen JA.Soft and hard tissue response to photocrosslinked poly(propylene fumarate) scaffolds in a rabbit model. *J Biomed Mater Res*. 2002; 59(3):547-56.

Fleming JE Jr, Cornell CN, Muschler GF. Bone cells and matrices in orthopedic tissue engineering.*Orthop Clin North Am*. 2000;31(3):357-74.

Friedenstein AJ, Chailakhjan RK, Lalykina KS. The development of fibroblast colonies in monolayer cultures of guinea-pig bone marrow and spleen cells. *Cell Tissue Kinet*. 1970; 3(4): 393-403.

Fu YC, Nie H, Ho ML, Wang CK, Wang CH. Optimized bone regeneration based on sustained release from three-dimensional fibrous PLGA/HAp composite scaffolds loaded with BMP-2. *Biotechnol Bioeng*. 2008; 99(4): 996-1006.

Gao TJ, Lindholm TS, Kommonen B, Ragni P, Paronzini A, Lindholm TC. Microscopic evaluation of bone-implant contact between hydroxyapatite, bioactive glass and tricalcium phosphate implanted in sheep diaphyseal defects. *Biomaterials* 1995; 16(15): 1175-9.

Gao TJ, Tuominen TK, Lindholm TS, Kommonen B, Lindholm TC. Morphological and biomechanical difference in healing in segmental tibial defects implanted with Biocoral or tricalcium phosphate cylinders. *Biomaterials* 1997; 18(3): 219-23.

Green SA, Jackson JM, Wall DM, Marinow H, Ishkanian J. Management of segmental defects by the Ilizarov intercalary bone transport method. *Clin Orthop Relat Res*. 1992; 280: 136-42.

Gugala Z, Gogolewski S. Regeneration of segmental diaphyseal defects in sheep tibiae using resorbable polymeric membranes: a preliminary study. *J Orthop Trauma* 1999; 13(3): 187-95.

Guo X, Zheng Q, Kulbatski I, Yuan Q, Yang S, Shao Z, Wang H, Xiao B, Pan Z, Tang S. Bone regeneration with active angiogenesis by basic fibroblast growth factor gene transfected mesenchymal stem cells seeded on porous beta-TCP ceramic scaffolds. *Biomed Mater*. 2006; 1(3): 93-9.

Hamidouche Z, Haÿ E, Vaudin P, Charbord P, Schüle R, Marie PJ, Fromigué O. FHL2 mediates dexamethasone-induced mesenchymal cell differentiation into osteoblasts by activating Wnt/β-catenin signaling-dependent Runx2 expression. *The FASEB Journal*. 2008; 22: 3813-22.

He Y, Zhang ZY, Zhu HG, Qiu W, Jiang X, Guo W. Experimental study on reconstruction of segmental mandible defects using tissue engineered bone combined bone marrow stromal cells with three-dimensional tricalcium phosphate. *J Craniofac Surg*. 2007; 18(4): 800-5.

Heise U, Osborn JF, Duwe F. Hydroxyapatite ceramic as a bone substitute. *International Orthopaedics* 1990; 14(3): 329-38.

Hench LL and Wilson J. An Introduction to Bioceramics. *Advanced Series in Ceramics - Vol 1, World Scientific*, USA, 1993, p.1-24.

Høl PJ, Mølster A, Gjerdet NR. Should the galvanic combination of titanium and stainless steel surgical implants be avoided? *Injury* 2008; 39(2): 161-9.

Hollinger JO, Brekke J, Gruskin E, Lee D. Role of bone substitutes. *Clin Orthop Relat Res*. 1996; 324: 55-65.

Holmes RE, Bone regeneration within a coralline hydroxyapatite implant. *Plast Reconstru Surg* 1979; 63: 626–633.

Hopp SG, Dahners LE, Gilbert JA. A study of the mechanical strength of long bone defects treated with various bone autograft substitutes: an experimental investigation in the rabbit. *J Orthop Res*. 1989; 7(4): 579-84.

Horwitz EM, Le Blanc K, Dominici M, Mueller I, Slaper-Cortenbach I, Marini FC, Deans RJ, Krause DS, Keating A; International Society for Cellular Therapy.Clarification of the nomenclature for MSC: The International Society for Cellular Therapy position statement. *Cytotherapy*. 2005;7(5):393-5.

Ishida H, Bellows CG, Aubin JE, Heersche JN. Characterization of the 1,25-(OH)2D3-induced inhibition of bone nodule formation in long-term cultures of fetal rat calvaria cells. *Endocrinology*. 1993; 132(1):61-6.

Isobe M, Yamazaki Y, Mori M, Amagasa T. Bone regeneration produced in rat femur defects by polymer capsules containing recombinant human bone morphogenetic protein-2. *J Oral Maxillofac Surg*. 1999; 57(6): 695-8.

Jackson MR. Fibrin sealants in surgical practice: An overview. *Am J Surg*. 2001; 182(2 Suppl): 1S-7S.

John A, Nair MB, Varma HK, Bernhardt A, Gelinsky M. Biodegradation and cytocompatibility studies of a triphasic ceramic coated porous hydroxyapatite for bone substitute applications. *Int. J. Appl. Ceram. Technol*. 2008; 5: 11–19.

Kadyala S, Jaiswal N, Bruder SP. Culture-expanded, bone marrow-derived mesenchymal stem cells can regenerate a critical-sized segmental bone defect. *Tissue Eng*. 1997, 3(2): 173-85.

Kehr H, Graftiaux AG, Gosset F, Bogorin I, Bencheikh K. Coral as graft in cervical spinal surgery. *Orthop Traumatol* 1993; 3: 287–293.

Kern S, Eichler H, Stoeve J, Klüter H, Bieback K. Comparative analysis of mesenchymal stem cells from bone marrow, umbilical cord blood, or adipose tissue. *Stem Cells*. 2006; 24(5): 1294-301.

Kitoh H, Kitakoji T, Tsuchiya H, Katoh M, Ishiguro N. Transplantation of culture expanded bone marrow cells and platelet rich plasma in distraction osteogenesis of the long bones. *Bone* 2007; 40(2): 522-8.

Kitoh H, Kitakoji T, Tsuchiya H, Mitsuyama H, Nakamura H, Katoh M, Ishiguro N. Transplantation of marrow-derived mesenchymal stem cells and platelet-rich plasma during distraction osteogenesis-a preliminary result of three cases. *Bone* 2004; 35(4): 892-8.

Komlev VS, Peyrin F, Mastrogiacomo M, Cedola A, Papadimitropoulos A, Rustichelli F, Cancedda R. Kinetics of in vivo bone deposition by bone marrow stromal cells into porous calcium phosphate scaffolds: an X-ray computed microtomography study. *Tissue Eng*. 2006; 12(12): 3449-58.

Kon E, Muraglia A, Corsi A, Bianco P, Marcacci M, Martin I, Boyde A, Ruspantini I, Chistolini P, Rocca M, Giardino R, Cancedda R, Quarto R. Autologous bone marrow stromal cells loaded onto porous hydroxyapatite ceramic accelerate bone repair in critical-size defects of sheep long bones. *J Biomed Mater Res*. 2000; 49(3): 328-37.

Kroeze RJ, Knippenberg M, Helder MN. Osteogenic differentiation strategies for adipose-derived mesenchymal stem cells.*Methods Mol Biol.* 2011; 702:233-48.

Kuznetsov SA, Mankani MH, Gronthos S, Satomura K, Bianco P, Robey PG.Circulating skeletal stem cells. *J. Cell Biol.* 2001; 153: 1133–1140.

Landesberg R, Moses M, Karpatkin M. Risks of using platelet rich plasma gel. *J Oral Maxillofac Surg.* 1998; 56(9): 1116-7.

Landesberg R, Roy M, Glickman RS. Quantification of growth factor levels using a simplified method of platelet-rich plasma gel preparation. *J Oral Maxillofac Surg*. 2000; 58(3): 297-300.

Langer R, Vacanti JP. *Tissue Engineering. Science* 1993; 260(5110):920-6.

Le Guéhennec L, Layrolle P, Daculsi G. A review of bioceramics and fibrin sealant. *Eur Cell Mater*. 2004; 8: 1-10.

Leskela HV, Risteli J, Niskanen S, Koivunen J, Ivaska KK, Lehenkari P (2003) Osteoblast recruitment from stem cells does not decrease by age at late adulthood. *Biochem Biophys Res Commun* 311:1008–1013.

Li Z, Yang Y, Wang C, Xia R, Zhang Y, Zhao Q, Liao W, Wang Y, Lu J. Repair of sheep metatarsus defects by using tissue-engineering technique. *J Huazhong Univ Sci Technolog Med Sci.* 2005; 25(1): 62-7.

Liu G, Zhao L, Zhang W, Cui L, Liu W, Cao Y. Repair of goat tibial defects with bone marrow stromal cells and beta-tricalcium phosphate. *J Mater Sci Mater Med.* 2008; 19(6): 2367-76.

Lucarelli E, Fini M, Beccheroni A, Giavaresi G, Di Bella C, Aldini NN, Guzzardella G, Martini L, Cenacchi A, Di Maggio N, Sangiorgi L, Fornasari PM, Mercuri M, Giardino R, Donati D. Stromal stem cells and platelet-rich plasma improve bone allograft integration. *Clin Orthop Relat Res*. 2005; 435: 62-8.

Maehata Y, Takamizawa S, Ozawa S, Kato Y, Sato S, Kubota E, Hata R. Both direct and collagen-mediated signals are required for active vitamin D3-elicited differentiation of human osteoblastic cells: roles of osterix, an osteoblast-related transcription factor. *Matrix Biol.* 2006; 25(1): 47-58.

Malgieri A, Kantzari E, Patrizi MP, Gambardella S. Bone marrow and umbilical cord blood human mesenchymal stem cells: state of the art.Int *J Clin Exp Med.* 2010;3(4):248-69.

Marcacci M, Kon E, Zaffagnini S, Giardino R, Rocca M, Corsi A, Benvenuti A, Bianco P, Quarto R, Martin I, Muraglia A, Cancedda R. Reconstruction of extensive long-bone defects in sheep using porous hydroxyapatite sponges. *Calcif Tissue Int.* 1999; 64(1): 83-90.

Martinez ME, del Campo MT, Medina S, Sanchez M, Sanchez-Cabezudo MJ, Esbrit P, Martinez P, Moreno I, Rodrigo A, Garces MV, Munuera L. Influence of skeletal site of origin and donor age on osteoblastic cell growth and differentiation. *Calcif Tissue Int* 1999; 64:280–286.

Marx RE, Carlson ER, Eichstaedt RM, Schimmele SR, Strauss JE, Georgeff KR. Platelet-rich plasma: Growth factor enhancement for bone grafts. *Oral Surg Oral Med Oral Pathol Oral Radiol Endod*. 1998; 85(6): 638-46.

Marx RE. Platelet-Rich Plasma (PRP): What is PRP and what is Not PRP? *Implant Dent.* 2001; 10(4): 225-8.

Mastrogiacomo M, Corsi A, Francioso E, Di Comite M, Monetti F, Scaglione S, Favia A, Crovace A, Bianco P, Cancedda R. Reconstruction of extensive long bone defects in sheep using bioresorbable bioceramics based on silicon stabilized Tricalcium phosphate. *Tissue Eng*. 2006; 12(5): 1261-73.

Mauney JR, Volloch V, Kaplan DL. Role of adult mesenchymal stem cells in bone tissue engineering applications: current status and future prospects. *Tissue Eng*. 2005; 11(5-6): 787-802.

Meana A, Iglesias J, Del Rio M, Larcher F, Madrigal B, Fresno MF, Martin C, San Roman F, Tevar F. Large surface of cultured human epithelium obtained on a dermal matrix based on live fibroblast-containing fibrin gels. *Burns* 1998; 24(7): 621-30.

Mooren RE, Merkx MA, Bronkhorst EM, Jansen JA, Stoelinga PJ. The effect of platelet-rich plasma on early and late bone healing: an experimental study in goats. *Int J Oral Maxillofac Surg*. 2007; 36(7): 626-31.

Morsi E. Tibial reconstruction using a non-vascularised fibular transfer. *Int Orthop.* 2002; 26(6): 377-80.

Muschler GF, Boehm C, Easley K. Aspiration to obtain osteoblast progenitor cells from human bone marrow: the influence of aspiration volume. *J Bone Joint Surg Am.* 1997; 79(11):1699-709.

Muschler GF, Nitto H, Boehm CA, Easley KA.Age- and gender-related changes in the cellularity of human bone marrow and the prevalence of osteoblastic progenitors.*J Orthop Res*. 2001 Jan;19(1):117-25.

Nair MB, Suresh Babu S, Varma HK, John A. A triphasic ceramic-coated porous hydroxyapatite for tissue engineering application. *Acta Biomater*. 2008; 4(1):173-81.

Nair MB, Varma H, Shenoy SJ, John A. Treatment of goat femur segmental defects with silica-coated hydroxyapatite--one-year follow-up. *Tissue Eng Part A*. 2010; 16(2):385-91.

Nair MB, Varma HK, John A. Platelet-rich plasma and fibrin glue coated bioactive ceramics enhances growth and differentiation of goat bone marrow-derived stem cells. *Tissue Eng Part A*. 2009a; 15(7):1619-31.

Nair MB, Varma HK, John A. Triphasic ceramic coated hydroxyapatite as a niche for goat stem cell-derived osteoblasts for bone regeneration and repair. *J Mater Sci Mater Med*. 2009b; 20 Suppl 1:S251-8.

Nair MB, Varma HK, Menon KV, Shenoy SJ, John A. The reconstruction of goat femur segmental defect using triphasic ceramic coated hydroxyapatite together with autologous cells and platelet-rich plasma. *Acta Biomater*. 2009c; 5(5):1742-55.

Nair MB, Varma HK, Menon KV, Shenoy SJ, John A. Tissue regeneration and repair of goat segmental femur defect with bioactive triphasic ceramic-coated hydroxyapatite scaffold. *J Biomed Mater Res A*. 2009d; 91(3):855-65.

Nakahara H, Dennis JE, Bruder SP, Haynesworth SE, Lennon DP, Caplan AI. In vitro differentiation of bone and hypertrophic cartilage from periosteal-derived cells.*Exp Cell Res*. 1991; 195(2):492-503.

Nemmar A, Nemery B, Hoet PH, Van Rooijen N, Hoylaerts MF. Silica particles enhance peripheral thrombosis: key role of lung macrophage-neutrophil cross-talk. Am *J Respir Crit Care Med*. 2005; 171(8): 872-9.

Neuhuber B, Swanger SA, Howard L, Mackay A, Fischer I. Effects of plating density and culture time on bone marrow stromal cell characteristics. *Exp Hematol*. 2008; 36(9):1176-85.

Nikolidakis D, van den Dolder J, Wolke JG, Stoelinga PJ, Jansen JA. The effect of platelet-rich plasma on the bone healing around calcium phosphate-coated and non-coated oral implants in trabecular bone. *Tissue Eng*. 2006; 12(9): 2555-63.

Nishida S, Endo N, Yamagiwa H, Tanizawa T, Takahashi HE (1999) Number of osteoprogenitor cells in human bone marrow markedly decreases after skeletal maturation. *J Bone Miner Metab* 17:171–177.

Nordström EG, Sánchez Muñoz OL. Physics of bone bonding mechanism of different surface bioactive ceramic materials in vitro and in vivo. *Biomed Mater Eng*. 2001; 11(3): 221-31.

Pietak AM, Reid JW, Stott MJ, Sayer M. Silicon substitution in the calcium phosphate bioceramics. *Biomaterials* 2007; 28(28): 4023-32.

Rai B, Oest ME, Dupont KM, Ho KH, Teoh SH, Guldberg RE. Combination of platelet-rich plasma with polycaprolactone-tricalcium phosphate scaffolds for segmental bone defect repair. *J Biomed Mater Res*. A 2007; 81(4): 888-99.

Reichert JC, Saifzadeh S, Wullschleger ME, Epari DR, Schütz MA, Duda GN, Schell H, van Griensven M, Redl H, Hutmacher DW.The challenge of establishing preclinical models for segmental bone defect research. *Biomaterials*. 2009; 30(12):2149-63.

Schlegel KA, Donath K, Rupprecht S, Falk S, Zimmermann R, Felszeghy E, Wiltfang J. De novo bone formation using bovine collagen and platelet-rich plasma. *Biomaterials* 2004; 25(23): 5387-93.

Seong JM, Kim BC, Park JH, Kwon IK, Mantalaris A, Hwang YS. Stem cells in bone tissue engineering.*Biomed Mater*. 2010; 5(6):062001.

Shimazaki K, Mooney V. Comparative study of porous hydroxyapatite and tricalcium phosphate as bone substitute. *J Orthop Res*. 1985; 3(3): 301-10.

Sierra DH. Fibrin sealant adhesive systems: A review of their chemistry, material properties and clinical applications. *J Biomater Appl*. 1993; 7(4): 309-52.

Singh R, Dahotre NB. Corrosion degradation and prevention by surface modification of biometallic materials. *J Mater Sci Mater Med*. 2007; 18(5): 725-51.

Son E, Do H, Joo HM, Pyo S. Induction of alkaline phosphatase activity by L-ascorbic acid in human osteoblastic cells: a potential role for CK2 and Ikaros. *Nutrition* 2007; 23(10): 745-53.

Sporn LA, Bunce LA, Francis CW. Cell proliferation on fibrin: modulation by fibrinopeptide cleavage. Blood 1995; 86(5): 1802-10.

Stenderup K, Justesen J, Clausen C, Kassem M (2003) Aging is associated with decreased maximal life span and accelerated senescence of bone marrow stromal cells. *Bone* (NY) 33:919– 926.

Sugiura F, Kitoh H and Ishiguro N. Osteogenic potential of rat mesenchymal stem cells after several passages. *Biochem Biophys Res Commun*. 2004; 316(1): 233-9.

Tachibana Y, Ninomiya S, Kim YT, Sekikawa M. Tissue response to porous hydroxyapatite ceramic in the human femoral head. *J Orthop Sci*. 2003; 8(4): 549-53.

Ter Brugge PJ, Jansen JA. In vitro osteogenic differentiation of rat bone marrow cells subcultured with and without dexamethasone. *Tissue Eng*. 2002; 8(2): 321-31.

Tomford WW. Transmission of disease through transplantation of musculoskeletal allografts. *J Bone Joint Surg Am*. 1995; 77(11): 1742-54.

Tomić S, Bumbasirević M, Lesić A, Mitković M, Atkinson HD. Ilizarov frame fixation without bone graft for atrophic humeral shaft nonunion: 28

patients with a minimum 2-year follow-up. *J Orthop Trauma*. 2007; 21(8): 549-56.

Wall ME, Bernacki SH, Loboa EG. Effects of serial passaging on the adipogenic and osteogenic differentiation potential of adipose-derived human mesenchymal stem cells. *Tissue Eng*. 2007; 13(6): 1291-8.

Wang M. Developing bioactive composite materials for tissue replacement. *Biomaterials* 2003; 24(13): 2133-51.

Weibrich G, Kleis WK, Hafner G, Hitzler WE, Wagner W. Comparison of platelet, leukocyte, and growth factor levels in point-of-care platelet-enriched plasma, prepared using a modified Curasan kit, with preparations received from a local blood bank. *Clin Oral Implants Res*. 2003; 14(3): 357-62.

Wheeler DL and Enneking WF, Allograft bone decreases in strength in vivo over time. *Clin Orthop Relat Res* 2005; 435: 36–42.

Wippermann B, Donow C, Schratt HE, den Boer FC, Blokhuis T, Patka P. The influence of hydroxyapatite granules on the healing of a segmental defect filled with autologous bone marrow. *Ann Chir Gynaecol*. 1999; 88(3): 194-7.

Yamada Y, Seong Boo J, Ozawa R, Nagasaka T, Okazaki Y, Hata K, Ueda M. Bone regeneration following injection of mesenchymal stem cells and fibrin glue with a biodegradable scaffold. *J Craniomaxillofac Surg*. 2003; 31(1): 27-33.

Yamada Y, Ueda M, Naiki T, Takahashi M, Hata K, Nagasaka T. Autogenous injectable bone for regeneration with mesenchymal stem cells and platelet-rich plasma: tissue-engineered bone regeneration. *Tissue Eng*. 2004; 10(5-6): 955-64.

Yuan J, Cui L, Zhang WJ, Liu W, Cao Y. Repair of canine mandibular bone defects with bone marrow stromal cells and porous beta-tricalcium phosphate. *Biomaterials* 2007; 28(6): 1005-13.

Zhu L, Liu W, Cui L, Cao Y. Tissue-engineered bone repair of goat-femur defects with osteogenically induced bone marrow stromal cells. *Tissue Eng*. 2006; 12(3): 423-33.

Zur Nieden NI, Kempka G, Ahr HJ. In vitro differentiation of embryonic stem cells into mineralized osteoblasts. *Differentiation* 2003; 71(1): 18-27.

In: Induced Stem Cells
Editors: P. Sullivan and E. Mortensen
ISBN: 978-1-61324-613-9

Chapter III

Induced Pluripotent Stem Cell-Derived Hepatocytes as an Alternative to Human Adult Hepatocytes

Takeshi Katsuda[1,2], Yasuyuki Sakai[2] and Takahiro Ochiya[1]
[1]Division of Molecular and Cellular Medicine, National Cancer Center Research Institute, Tokyo, Japan
[2]Institute of Industrial Science (IIS), The University of Tokyo, Tokyo, Japan

Abstract

Recent advances in induced pluripotent stem (iPS) cell research have attracted much attention. The ability to generate such cells from somatic cells has implications for overcoming both immunological rejection and the ethical issues associated with embryonic stem (ES) cells. Hepatocytes derived from patient-specific iPS cells offer a possible solution to the shortage of cell sources in cell replacement therapy, drug screening, and disease model. Despite such great promise, however, recent articles have questioned the viability of the therapeutic applications of iPS cells. These cells must, therefore, satisfy stringent criteria prior to practical use. The main focus of this review is a description of the current status of hepatic differentiation technology of iPS cells and a discussion of the concerns regarding the practical use of these techniques in cell replacement therapy, drug screening, and disease model. The current status of strategies for generating iPS cells and the accumulated knowledge on strategies for differentiating ES cells into hepatocytes will be summarized. We also refer to the possibility of direct conversion of adult somatic cells into functional hepatocytes.

1. Introduction

An alternative cell source for functional hepatocytes has been essential for various applications in medicine. For severe liver failures, orthotopic liver transplantation is the only effective treatment, but it is currently limited by donor shortage. This has led to the development of cell replacement therapy in the form of hepatocyte transplantation and artificial liver support devices [1,2]. However, these approaches have been confronted with the serious problem of obtaining hepatocytes in sufficient amounts and quality. Researchers in the field of drug screening have also been presented with a donor shortage problem. In drug screening, primary human hepatocytes are the current gold-standard because they express the entire complement of drug metabolizing enzymes and transporters [3]. However, this approach is hindered by the low quality of isolated hepatocytes. Generally, isolated hepatocytes are available only from cadaveric donor livers; thus the cells largely lack quality and quantity [4]. These situations have led researchers on a quest for alternative cell sources that can generate hepatic cells with the ability to proliferate *in vitro* and that can express hepatic functions.

Human embryonic stem (ES) cells which are capable of indefinitely proliferating and differentiating into any adult cell types have, therefore, been extensively studied [5,6]. Accordingly, many reports have shown that ES cells can be differentiated into functional hepatocytes *in vivo* and *in vitro* [7]. Furthermore, ES cells exhibit another beneficial aspect, namely, that they can also serve as a cell source for modeling genetic liver diseases. Since ES cells can go through embryonic and postembryonic development, they have the possibility to recapitulate the pathology of genetic diseases. Thus, human ES cells have raised expectations among researchers and the general public alike.

However, the use of ES cells has inherent problems. Ethical controversies regarding the use of human embryos, as well as immune rejection problems following transplantation, have hindered the applications of human ES cells. In addition, despite great efforts to generate human ES cells harboring disease-specific mutations as disease models in many laboratories, this strategy has faced challenges because of the inefficient methods to genetically modify ES cells [8].

The recent breakthrough in stem cell research has opened up new possibilities for solving these issues. Yamanaka and his colleagues demonstrated that retroviral transduction of a defined set of transcription factors give rise to induced pluripotent stem (iPS) cells directly from fibroblast cultures [9,10]. After their discoveries, remarkable progress has continued at a rapid pace, raising hopes that iPS cell technology will pave the way for cell replacement therapy, drug screening, and disease model. In addition to the possibility of circumventing immune rejection and ethical issues, derivation of patient-specific iPS cells for various liver diseases implies useful platforms for drug discovery and studying the mechanisms of diseases.

One of the major hurdles for achieving these goals is to establish an efficient protocol for differentiating iPS cells to functional hepatocytes. During the past decade, a great deal of knowledge has been accumulated regarding *in vitro* differentiation of ES cells to hepatic cell lineages, and recently researchers have demonstrated that the methods gained from that knowledge is applicable to differentiation of iPS cells into hepatic cells. Moreover, hepatocytes derived from patient-specific iPS cells have been found to recapitulate key pathological features of the diseases affecting the patients from which they were derived.

In this review, we will first summarize the current status of strategies for generating iPS cells, and then overview strategies for differentiating ES cells into hepatocytes. Subsequently we will describe the latest reports on hepatic differentiation of iPS cells including patient-specific ones. We will also discuss the concerns regarding the practical use of iPS cells in cell replacement therapy, drug screening, and disease model. In the last section, we will refer to the possibility of direct conversion of somatic cells into functional hepatocytes.

2. Generation of Pluripotent Stem Cells from Somatic Cells

The discovery that mouse and human somatic cells can be reprogrammed to pluripotent stem cells has created enthusiasm for their potential applications in regenerative medicine. Takahashi and Yamanaka first reported that transduction of a defined set of transcription factors, Kruppel-like factor 4 (KLF4), Octamer 3/4 (OCT4), SRY box–containing protein 2 (SOX2), and c-Myc, gave rise to iPS cells directly from mouse fibroblasts [9]. These cells were similar to ES cells in morphology, proliferation, the expression of some ES cell marker genes, and teratoma formation. Despite the similarity, however, they were not identical to ES cells, and failed to produce adult chimeric mice. In 2007, mouse iPS cells capable of germline transmission were generated [11-13], and human iPS cells were generated from fibroblasts [10,14,15].

In the several years since those first generation iPS cells were reported, remarkable progress has continued at a rapid pace in the development of reprogramming methods. Nakagawa *et al.* generated mouse and human iPS cells without transduction of Myc, which indicated reduction of the tumorigenesis risk [16]. In 2009, Kim *et al.* generated iPS cells from mouse neural stem cells by retroviral transduction of OCT4 alone [17]. Thereafter, several reports have shown that iPS cells can be generated even without viral integration. These methods involve transient expression of reprogramming factors using plasmids [18], administration of synthetic mRNA [19], lentiviruses or transposons followed by transgene removal using Cre-mediated excision or re-expression of transposase [20,21]. As another novel strategy, several reports have shown that reprogramming factors could be replaced by identified chemicals, such as histone deacetylase inhibitors and MEK inhibitors [22,23].

Such remarkable progress has significantly implies that the generation of patient-specific iPS cells holds great promise for cell replacement therapy, drug screening, and disease model (Figure 1). For the practical application of iPS cell technology to these fields, directly differentiating iPS cells into cell types of interest is crucial. It has already been shown that iPS cells can be differentiated *in vitro* into various cell types including neural progenitors, motor neurons, domapinergic neurons, retinal cells, adipocytes, endothelial cells, fibroblasts and hepatocytes [8]. Importantly, some of these reports involve the generation of patient-specific iPS cells, indicating promise for the future use of iPS cell technology in medicine. In the next two sections, we will focus on the generation of hepatocytes from pluripotent stem cells, namely, ES cells as well as iPS cells, and discuss the feasibility of those technologies to alternate use of human hepatocytes.

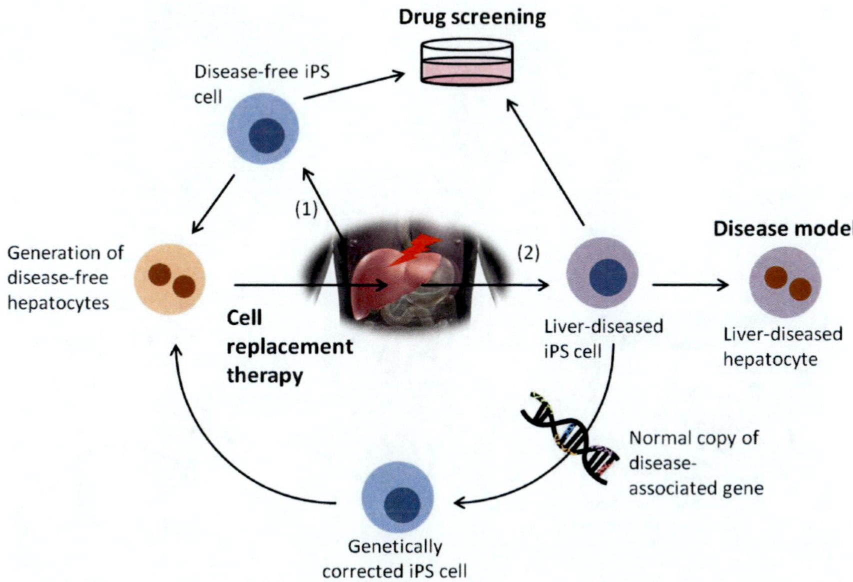

Figure 1. Possible application of patient-specific iPS cells. (1) In case of a non-genetic liver disease, generated iPS cells are disease-free, thus can be directly differentiated into hepatocytes and used for cell replacement therapy as well as drug screening. (2) In case of a genetic liver disease, reprogrammed iPS cells can be used for disease model and drug screening. For cell replacement therapy, the defect of such iPS cells should be corrected by introduction of the wild-type gene. Resultant genetically corrected iPS cells can be differentiated into hepatocytes and used for cell replacement therapy.

3. Overview of Generation of Hepatocytes from ES Cells

Prior to reviewing the current status of the generation of hepatocytes from iPS cells, we will overview the methodology for differentiating ES cells into hepatocytes. Theoretically, pluripotent stem cells including ES and iPS cells can precisely trace the process of *in vivo* liver development. Thus, researchers have attempted to direct these cells to hepatocytes *in vitro* by recapitulating the *in vivo* environment that hepatic precursors experience. In this section we will first mention the development of the liver. All these processes are illustrated in Figure 2. Then we will overview the representative protocols for differentiating ES cells to hepatocytes.

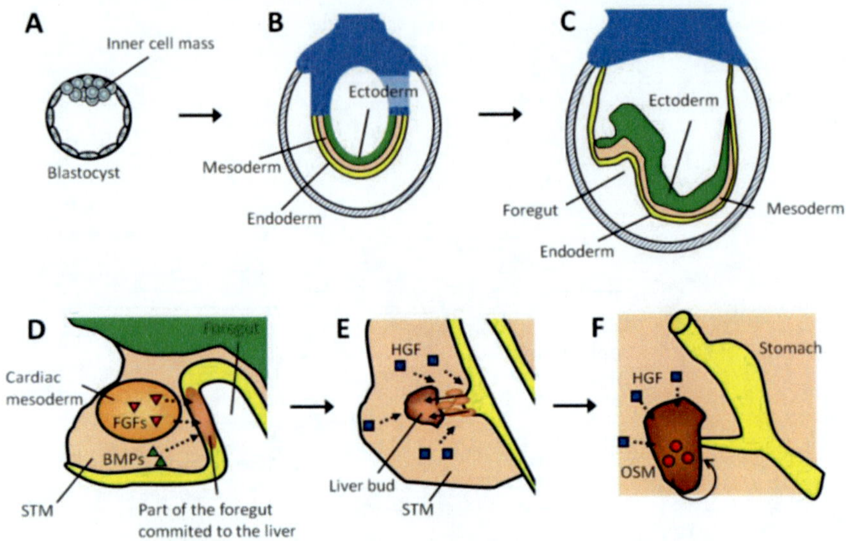

Figure 2. Summary of liver development. (A) The blastocyst harbors the inner cell mass that derives ES cells. (B) During late postimplantation, the epiblast gives rise to three germ layers — ectoderm, mesoderm, and endoderm. (C) The foregut is formed under the regulation of transcription factors such as FOXA2 and GATA4. (D) Part of the foregut generates the liver bud, the primordial diverticulum that gives rise to the liver parenchyma. FGFs from the cardiac mesoderm and BMPs from the STM cooperatively specify the liver fate in the foregut endoderm. (E) As hepatoblasts proliferate and migrate into the STM, the liver diverticulum becomes thicker to form the liver bud. HGF that is expressed in the STM, hepatoblasts, and endothelial cells surrounding the liver bud plays a critical role in the outgrowth of the liver bud. (F) OSM, in a paracrine manner, induces the differentiation of immature hepatocytes to functional hepatocytes of the neonatal liver. HGF is also implicated in hepatocyte differentiation.

3.1. Development of the Liver

Liver development initiates from the endoderm. During late postimplantation, the epiblast gives rise to three germ layers — ectoderm, mesoderm, and endoderm. Nodal, a member of the TGFβ superfamily, is essential for formation of the mesoderm and endoderm during gastrulation in mice and humans [24]. High levels of Nodal signaling specify definitive endoderm and lower levels of Nodal signaling specify mesoderm [25,26]. Subsequently, transcription factors forkhead box A (FOXA)2/hepatocyte neculear factor (HNF)3β and GATA binding protein (GATA)4, which are expressed in definitive endoderm, regulate morphogenesis of the foregut [27,28].

Part of the foregut generates the liver bud, the primordial diverticulum that gives rise to the liver parenchyma. Fibroblast growth factors (FGFs) from the cardiac mesoderm and bone morphogenic proteins (BMPs) from the septum transversum mesenchyme (STM) cooperatively specify the liver fate in the foregut endoderm [29,30]. Subsequently, the foregut endoderm forms the liver diverticulum, in which multipotent endoderm cells are committed to liver progenitor cells called hepatoblasts [31]. Hepatoblasts have the capacity to differentiate into hepatocytes that compose the liver parenchyma and the cholangiocyte lining the bile ducts. As hepatoblasts proliferate and migrate into the STM, the liver diverticulum becomes thicker to form the liver bud [32]. Hepatocyte growth factor (HGF) that is expressed in STM, hepatoblasts, and endothelial cells surrounding the liver bud plays a critical role in the outgrowth of the liver bud [33, 34].

Oncostatin M (OSM), in combination with a glucocorticoid such as dexamethasone (DEX), directs hepatoblasts to differentiate into hepatocytes, and then induces hepatic maturation [35]. OSM, an interleukin-6 family cytokine, is a paracrine factor produced by hematopoietic cells. In contrast to the adult liver, the fetal liver lacks metabolic functions. Instead, it supports the hematopoietic function, which afterward shifts to the bone marrow and the spleen. Like OSM, HGF in the presence of DEX also induces hepatic differentiation and maturation [36]. The fetal liver acquires various additional metabolic functions near birth, and full functions after birth.

3.2. Strategy for Commitment of ES Cells into Hepatocytes

In the last decade, *in vitro* differentiation of ES cells to hepatocytes has been explored by mimicking the liver development process. Most protocols consist of these three steps: directing undifferentiated ES cells into the definitive endoderm (step 1), differentiation of the endodermal cells into liver progenitor cells (step 2), and specification of the liver progenitors to hepatocytes and subsequent maturation (step 3). Here, we overview the representative protocols for induction of hepatocytes from ES cells. Details are summarized in Table 1.

Table 1. Protocols for commitment of ES cells into hepatocytes

Species	Differentiation protocol	Hepatic markers/functions	Ref.
Mouse	EB formation / FGF1 / HGF / OSM + DEX + ITS	ALB, G6P, TAT, TTR, AAT	37
Mouse	EB formation / FGF1 + FGF2 / HGF / OSM + DEX + ITS	ALB, AFP, TAT, Urea synthesis	38
Mouse	EB formation / plated onto petridish	AFP, ALB, HNF4α, Transfferin	39
Mouse	EB formation / plated onto gelatin-coated plate	AFP, ALB, TTR, AAT, TDO2, CPS1, PEPCK, LST1, FOXA2, ICG uptake	40
Mouse	EB formation / plated onto tissue culture plate	AFP, ALB, TTR, AAT, G6P, GST, FOXA1/2/3	41
Mouse	EB formation / plated onto gelatin-coated plate, RA + HGF + NGFβ	ALB, G6P, TTR, HNF4α, AAT	42
Mouse	EB formation, ActA / FACS sorting, BMP4 + FGF2 + Activin A	FOXA2, ALB, AFP, TAT, CPS1, CYP7A1, CYP3A11, ALB production, PAS staining	43
Mouse	EB formation / ActA + FGF2 / co-cultured with human nonparenchymal liver cell lines, dHGF + DMSO / DEX	ALB, CK18, TAT, G6P, FOXA2, HNF4α, CYP7A1, CK19, AFP, ammonia detoxification, glucose production, metabolism of lidocaine and diazepam	44
Mouse	Monolayer on gelatin-coated plate, RA / passaged onto collagen-coated plate, HGF + FGF1 + FGF4 / OSM + DEX	ALB, TTR, TAT, G6P, TDO2, CK8, LST1, CPS1, PEPCK, CYP1A1, FOXA2, HNF4α, CK18, ALB, fibrinogen synthesis	45
Human	Monolayer / ActA / ActA + ITS / FGF4 + BMP2 / HGF /OSM + DEX	AFP, ALB, CK8, CK18, G6P, AAT, HNF4α, PEPCK, TDO2, TAT, CYP7A1, CYP3A4, CYP2B6, LDL uptake, ICG uptake, PAS staining, PROD	46
Human	Monolayer / DMSO / HCM + HGF + EGF / HCM + HGF + OSM	AFP, ALB, AAT, TDO2, HNF4α, C/EBPα, TTR, Hepar 1, CYP3A4 activity, PAS staining, ICG uptake and excretion	47
Human	Monolayer on matrigel-coated plate, SB + ActA / passaged onto matrigel-coated plate, DMSO / HGF + OSM	AFP, ALB, TAT, TDO2, TTR, CAR, ApoF, Pax6, c-Met, CK18, CK19, CYP2C9, CYP2C19, CYP2D6, CYP3A4, CYP3A7, PAS staining, CYP3A4 enzyme activity, fibrinoven, fibronectin, and α-2 macroglobulin production	48

AAT, α1-antitrypsin; ActA, activin A; ApoF, apolipoprotein F; CPS-1, carbamyl phosphate synthetase 1; EGF, epidermal growth factor; dHGF, HGF with deletion of 5 amino acids; GST, glutathione-S-transferase; ICC, immunocytochemistry; ITS, insulin-transferrin-selenium; LST1, liver specific organic anion transporter-1; PAS, periodic acid-Schiff; PEPCK, phosphoenolpyruvate carboxykinase; PROD, entoxyresorufin-O-dealkylas; RA, retinoic acid; SB, sodium butyrate; TTR, transthyretin

In the first step, undifferentiated ES cells are initially induced to the definitive endoderm. Mainly in classical protocols, embryoid bodies (EBs), which mimic the developing embryo, were formed to induce spontaneous differentiation of ES cells [37-44]. Formed EBs were plated onto plastic dishes coated with an extracellular matrix such as collagen or gelatin. Then, the differentiation process proceeded to the subsequent step, or the cells underwent further endodermal induction by the addition of exogenous factors. While EB formation is useful for inducing an efficient differentiation of ES cells, the resultant cells show a mixed population of three germ layers. Thus, in other protocols, ES cells have been cultured as a monolayer in the presence of exogenous inducers for direct differentiation into the endoderm [45-48]. High concentrations of activin A, a TGFβ family member that binds the same receptors as endogenous endoderm inducer Nodal, have been used [49,50]. Generated endodermal cells have been generally characterized by the expression of FOXA2, SOX17, and GATA4.

In the second step, induced endodermal cells undergo subsequent treatment for specification to hepatic progenitor cells. FGF1, FGF2 and FGF4, and BMP2 and BMP4, which are respectively secreted from the cardiac mesoderm and the STM *in vivo*, have been added for hepatic specification *in vitro* [37, 38, 43-46]. In addition, HGF, which is expressed in the STM and the liver nonparenchymal cells, has been used [37,38,42,44-47]. In this step, hepatic progenitor cells have been characterized mainly by the expression of alpha-fetoprotein (AFP), which is an early fetal hepatic marker, and its expression decreases as the liver develops [51].

Finally, in the third step, hepatic progenitor cells are specified to hepatocytes, and undergo a maturation process. To induce proliferation and differentiation, HGF has been used [37,38,42,43-47]. OSM has also been used for hepatocyte differentiation and further maturation to derive the functions of hepatocytes [37,38,45-48]. In addition, dexamethasone, a synthetic glucocorticoid, has been used to induce the enzyme activity of hepatocytes such as glucose-6-phosphatase (G6P), tyrosine aminotransferase (TAT), and cytochrome P450 (CYP)s [37,38,44-46]. Mature hepatocytes have been characterized mainly by the expression of albumin (ALB), tryptophan 2,3-dioxygenase (TDO2) and TAT.

4. Generation of Hepatocytes from iPS Cells

4.1. Current Status of Research on Hepatic Differentiation of iPS Cells

Recently, researchers have confirmed that iPS cells can be differentiated into authentic hepatocytes by *in vivo* experiments. Si-Tayeb *et al.*, by examining embryos derived solely from mouse iPS cells by tetraploid complementation, first confirmed that iPS cells were competent to follow a hepatic developmental program that produced all liver cell lineages [53]. Espejel *et al.*, by generating chimeric mice in which all hepatocytes were iPS cell-derived, also confirmed that iPS cell–derived hepatocytes have the functional and proliferative capabilities needed for liver regeneration in mice [59]. Moreover, they demonstrated that fibroblast origin and reprogramming did not diminish the regenerative capabilities of iPS cell–derived hepatocytes by challenging 2/3 partial hepatectomy or transplantation into liver-diseased mice.

Meanwhile, an increasing number of reports have demonstrated that iPS cells can be directed into hepatocytes *in vitro*. Most of them have followed protocols that were established based on the knowledge regarding *in vitro* differentiation of ES cells to hepatocytes (Table 2). The majority of the protocols described involve a direct induction to differentiate into endoderm, hepatic progenitors, and mature hepatocytes using a stepwise differentiation method. Of these, Inamura *et al.* proposed a challenging method to generate hepatoblasts from human iPS cells by adenovirus-mediated overexpression of the HEX gene, a homeotic gene essential for hepatic differentiation [63]. Others include an initial step of EB formation and co-culture with supporting cells. Differentiated hepatocytes have been characterized by the expression of a panel of marker genes at the mRNA level and/or protein level. Their functionality has been confirmed by albumin secretion, urea secretion, glycogen storage, low-density lipoprotein (LDL) uptake, indocyanine green (ICG) uptake and release, and CYP activity. A more stringent test of the differentiation ability would be an *in vivo* functionality of the differentiated cells. Accordingly, Si-Tayeb *et al.* and Gai *et al.* demonstrated that iPS cell-derived hepatocytes had the inherent capacity to integrate into the hepatic parenchyma *in vivo* [53,56].

Table 2. Protocols for commitment of iPS cells into hepatocytes

Species/ origin	Differentiation protocol	CYP expression	Reference
Human / fibroblast	Adherent culture on MEF feeder cells, ActA / FGF4 + BMP2 / HGF + KGF / OSM + DEX / OSM + DEX + N2 + B27	2A6 (mRNA), 2B4 (enzyme activity), 3A4 (mRNA, ICC)	52
Human / foreskin fibroblast	Monolayer on matrigel-coated plate, ActA B27 / B27 + BMP4 + FGF2 / B27 + HGF, 4%-O_2 / OSM	Not detected.	53
Human / fibroblast	Monolayer on matrigel, ActA + Wnt3a / Act / DMSO / HGF + OSM	1A2, 3A4 (enzyme activitiy), 7A1 (mRNA)	54
Mouse / MEF	Monolayer on gelatin-coated plate, DMSO / SB	7A1 (mRNA)	55
Mouse / fibroblast	EB formation / plated onto matrigel-coated plate, ActA + Wnt3 / FGF2 + DMSO / HGF + DMSO / HGF + OSM + DEX	1A1 (ICC)	56
Human / hepatocyte	Monolayer, ActA / passaged onto collagen I-coated plate, FGF4 + HGF / FGF4 + HGF + OSM + DEX	1A2 (enzyme activity), 3A4 (ICC, enzyme activity)	57
Human / fibroblast	Monolayer, ActA + FGF2 + BMP4 / FGF10 / FGF10 + RA + SB431542 / FGF4 + HGF + EGF	Not determined.	58
Mouse / MEF	Generation of chimeric mice by injection of iPS cells into blastocysts obtained from FAH-deficient mice	Not determined.	59
Human / dermal fibrobalst	Monolayer, ActA + BMP4 / ActA + FGF2 + B27 / ActA / HGF + OSM	3A4 (enzyme activitiy)	60
Human / foreskin fibroblast	Co-cultured with human ES cell-deirved fibroblast like cells	7A1 (mRNA), ethoxyresorufin-O-deethylase activity	61
Human / skin fibroblast	EB formation / plated onto matrigel-coated plate, ActA / DMSO + HGF/ DEX	1A1 (ICC), 3A4 (mRNA), pentoxyresorufin O-dealkylase activity	62
Human / embryonic lung fibroblast	Monolayer on laminin-coated plate, ActA + FGF2 / BMP4 + FGF4 / adenoviral transduction of HEX, BMP4 + FGF4 / FGF4 + HGF + OSM + DEX	2D6, 7A1 (mRNA), 3A4 (mRNA, enzyme activity)	63
Mouse / MEF	EB formation / plated onto gelatin-coated plate, ActA + FGF2 / HGF	Not determined.	64
Mouse / bone marrow adherent cell	Monolayer on matrigel-coated plate, ActA + Wnt3a / BMP4 + FGF2 /FGF1 + FGF4 + FGF8 / HGF + Follistatin	3A7, 7A1 (mRNA), 1A2 (enzyme activity)	65
Human / fetal foreskin fibroblast	Monolayer, ActA + SB / DMSO / HGF + OSM	1A1, 2C9, 2E1, 2F1, 2C19, 11B2 (mRNA)	66

FAH, fumarylacetoacetate hydrolase; ICC, immunocytochemistry; KGF, keratinocyte growth factor; MEF, mouse embryonic fibroblast; N2, N2 supplement; B27, B27 supplement

4.2. Possibility of iPS Cells as a Cell Source for Cell Replacement Therapy

Applying stem cell technology to cell replacement therapy in liver diseases has long been desired, though it has not yet been realized. As alternatives to orthotopic liver transplantation, cell replacement therapy in the form of hepatocyte transplantation and artificial livers including extracorporeal and intracorporeal devices have been explored [2,67,68]. However, these approaches require a much larger amount of hepatocytes than currently available [68]. Therefore, researchers have aimed at obtaining transplantable cells from other sources such as ES cells, adult stem cells, or liver progenitor cells. Of these, ES cells have attracted the most attention since they provide an unlimited cell source owing to their infinite proliferative capacity. However, the clinical application of ES cells involves immune rejection after transplantation and ethical concerns regarding the use of human embryos.

iPS cells may be able to completely overcome the obstacles associated with human ES cells, thus the technology to generate hepatocytes from iPS cells has created enthusiasm for their potential applications in cell replacement therapy. In cases where a sporadic form of a disease is due to epigenetic alterations in the liver, iPS cells derived from somatic cells from non-hepatic tissues could be therapeutic, since the reprogramming process should reverse the disease causing the epigenetic modifications. In contrast, in cases where specific genotypes are the root cause of diseases (for example, Crigler-Najjar syndrome, Wilson's disease and tyrosinemia), reprogramming will not alleviate the problem. In such cases, the resultant iPS cell-derived hepatocytes may succumb to the same degenerative processes that occurred in the patient. If a genetic defect is known, utilizing gene therapy approaches could restore cellular function. Several reports have provided proof-of-concept that iPS cell technology can be used for the generation of disease-corrected, patient-specific cells [69-71]. Hanna *et al.* corrected the mutant gene of iPS cells derived from an anemic mouse, differentiated them into hematopoietic progenitors, and importantly, demonstrated that these cells ameliorated some pathological features after transplantation back into the mouse [69].

Another attempt to apply iPS cells to cell replacement therapy is the generation of organs derived from donor iPS cells, using a xenogenic environment. Kobayashi *et al.* generated interspecific chimeras by injecting mouse or rat iPS cells into rat or mouse blastocysts, respectively, and confirmed that iPS cells were able to contribute to xenogenic development between mouse and rat [72]. Notably, they found that rat wild-type iPS cells injected into Pdx-/- (pancreatogenesis-disabled) mouse blastocysts generated a normally functioning rat pancreas in Pdx1-/- mice. This finding allows us to expect that a blastocyst complementation of hepatogenesis-disabled large animals such as pigs with human iPS cells should be able to generate a whole functioning human liver. Despite the large concern about safety at this moment, the realization of such a strategy has the possibility to solve the current donor shortage problem in liver transplantation.

4.3. Possibility of iPS Cell-Derived Hepatocytes as a Cell Source for Drug Screening and *In Vitro* Hepatic Disease Model

The CYP superfamily plays a key role in the detoxification and metabolic activation of various endogenous and exogenous compounds, such as drugs, carcinogens, and environmental chemicals [73]. Therefore, in drug screening, it is crucial to induce CYP activity in iPS cell-derived hepatocytes. A majority of reports showed that iPS cell-derived hepatocytes express CYPs such as CYP1A1, 1A2, 2A6, 2B4, 2D6, 3A4, and 7A1 at mRNA and/or protein levels (Table 2). Furthermore, it was also demonstrated in several reports that iPS cell-derived hepatocytes exhibited the enzymatic activities of CYP1A2 and/or CYP3A4, which are the key enzymes in drug metabolism. However, as discussed in the next section, the levels of CYP activities of iPS cell-derived hepatocytes have not yet been sufficient for drug screening.

The technique of generating hepatocytes from patient-specific iPS cells could provide useful platforms for drug discovery and offer unprecedented insights into liver disease mechanisms. Rashid *et al.* and Ghodsizadeh *et al.* proved for the first time that it was possible to derive iPS cells from patients suffering from inherited metabolic disorders: alpha1-antitrypsin deficiency (A1ATD), familial hypercholesterolemia (FH), glycogen storage disease type 1a (GSD1a) [60], GSD1b, tyrosinemia, progressive familial hereditary cholestasis, and Crigler-Najjar syndrome [62] (Table 3). Importantly, Rashid *et al.* demonstrated that these disease-specific iPS cell-derived hepatocytes recapitulated key pathological features of the diseases, such as aggregation of misfolded α1-antitrypsin in the endoplasmic reticulum, deficient LDL receptor–mediated cholesterol uptake, and elevated lipid and glycogen accumulation [60]. These findings suggest that human iPS cells can be used to model a diverse range of inherited diseases in adult cells.

Table 3. Generation of liver disease-specific iPS cells and their hepatic differentiation

Phenotype of disease	Hepatic differentiation	Recapitulation of symptoms	Reference
α1-antitrypsin deficiency	Yes.	Yes. Aggregation of misfolded mutant α1-antitrypsin in the endoplasmic reticulum.	60
Glycogen storage disease type 1a	Yes.	Yes. Elevated cellular lipid and glycogen accumulation.	60
familial hypercholesterolemia	Yes.	Yes. Deficient LDL receptor–mediated cholesterol uptake.	60
Hereditary tyrosinemia type 1	Not determined.	Not determined.	60
Crigler-Najjar syndrome type 1	Not determined.	Not determined.	60
Tyrosinemia type 1	Yes.	Not determined.	62
Glycogen storage type 1b	Yes.	Not determined.	62
Progressive familial hereditary cholestasis	Not determined.	Not determined.	62
Crigler-Najjar Syndrome	Yes.	Not determined.	62

Generating hepatocyte-derived iPS cells is also crucial, since certain liver diseases involve acquired somatic mutations that occur only in the hepatocytes of patients and not in other cell types [74-78]. So far, human iPS cells have been produced mostly from mesoderm (fibroblasts and blood cells) [10,14,15,79,80] or ectoderm (keratinocytes and neural stem cells) [81,82]. Liu *et al.*, for the first time, generated human iPS cells from adult hepatocytes, and demonstrated that these cells were able to directly differentiate into definitive endoderm, hepatic progenitors, and mature hepatocytes [57]. In addition, their report offers an insight toward comprehensive comparative investigations of the quality of human iPS cells of different origins.

4.4. Comparison among ES Cell-Derived Hepatocytes, iPS Cell-Derived Hepatocytes, and Primary Hepatocytes

Some of the reports described above compared human iPS cell-derived hepatocytes with ES cell derived-hepatoyctes in liver-enriched gene expression and liver-specific functions. These reports indicated that iPS cells behave similarly to ES cells in endodermal induction in terms of morphological assessment and gene expression profiles [52,53]. In addition, the patterns and the levels of hepatic functions of human iPS cell-derived hepatocytes were similar to those of ES cell-derived hepatocytes [52,53,58]. Si-Tayeb *et al.* performed array analyses and demonstrated that iPS cell–derived hepatocytes expressed the same hepatocyte mRNA fingerprint that was found for human ES cell–derived hepatocytes [53].

Of note, however, the expression levels and functional levels of hepatic markers of iPS cell-derived hepatocytes were lower in most cases when compared with adult liver samples. Human iPS and ES cells expressed liver-enriched genes including α1-antitrypsin, TDO2, CYP2A6, CYP3A4, and phase I and phase II enzymes at lower levels than human hepatocytes [52,53]. Song *et al.* showed that the CYP activities of the differentiated human iPS and ES cells were nearly 30-fold lower than those of human hepatocytes either at basal level or after drug induction [52]. These results suggest that although hepatocyte-like cells derived from both human ES or iPS cells have differentiated to a state that supports many hepatic activities, they do not entirely recapitulate mature liver function. Therefore, it seems essential to improve the final maturation stage in order to allow ES and iPS cell-derived hepatocytes to acquire full hepatic functions.

5. Challenging Issues in Application of iPS Cell-Derived Hepatocytes

So far, we have reviewed the potential of iPS cell-derived hepatocytes as a promising cell source for cell replacement therapy, drug screening, and disease model. However, before their use, hurdles remain that need to be cleared. Here, we will mainly discuss the issues that challenge their therapeutic application. We will also discuss possible challenges to the application of iPS cells to drug screening as well as to disease model.

5.1. Cell Replacement Therapy

First, a therapeutic application of iPS cells involves the risk of teratoma formation. As with ES cells, even a small number of undifferentiated iPS cells can form a teratoma. In addition, recently, iPS cells have been demonstrated to develop teratoma more efficiently and faster than human ES cells [83]. Thus, for a cell replacement therapy, it is essential to establish a method to direct iPS cells to differentiated cells as thoroughly as possible. In particular, this issue is a serious problem in hepatocyte transplantation therapy, which requires an extremely large amount of hepatocytes [1].

Second, the generation of iPS cells involves genetic modification, which could possibly give rise to obstacles in several aspects. Most reprogramming methods have used retroviruses or lentiviruses, which involve transgene integration. Although transgenes are largely silenced in iPS cells, it is possible that reactivation of transgenes causes tumorigenesis. Furthermore, insertional mutagenesis which can occur after the integration of heterologous genetic material into the genome, significantly increases the risk of tumorigenesis. Even though it is possible to circumvent transgene integration for generating iPS cells [18-23], there remains the risk that such iPS cells may contain other genetic alterations such as integration of small plasmid fragments or chemically induced mutations [84]. Another problem in cell replacement therapy involving genetic correction of patient-specific iPS cells is the potential immunological consequences [85]. Autologous iPS cells are devoid of alloreactivity. However, the absence of the corrected gene products would preclude the induction of self-tolerance during T cell repertoire collection, which would cause a T cell attack against the autologous iPS cell derivatives.

Third, the molecular and cellular characteristics of iPS cells have not been fully understood, which might cause unpredictable accidents in a future clinical application. The criteria for quality control of generated iPS cells should be the similarities to ES cells, since ES cells are natural and authentic pluripotent stem cells. Although iPS cells have similarity to ES cells in their morphology, expression of important ES cell marker genes, and their ability to form teratomas, it remains unclear whether they have truly identical properties. Gene expression signatures and microRNA profiling have demonstrated iPS cells and ES cells to be distinguishable [86,87]. Several studies have also shown that iPS cells differ from ES cells epigenetically [88,89]. Pick *et al.* studied the imprinting gene expression pattern of multiple human iPS cells, and demonstrated that iPS cells exhibited the presence of genes that showed aberrant expression levels, namely biallelic expression of several imprinting genes [89]. Another concern is the variation in the safety of iPS cells. Miura *et al.* evaluated the teratoma-forming propensity of secondary neurospheres (SNS) generated from iPS cell lines derived from different tissues in different ways, and found that the teratoma-forming propensities of SNS varied significantly depending on the iPS cells' tissue of origin [90]. It will be important to correlate these differences with the ways these iPS cells behave, and answer questions such as which ones are more stable and which ones form tumors more efficiently. In addition, for any future clinical application of iPS cells it is crucial to further understand the molecular characteristics underlying their various propensities and their differences from ES cells.

5.2. Drug Screening

Drug screening also has hurdles to be cleared prior to practical use. The most serious problem is, as described in section 4.4, that hepatic functions of iPS cell-derived hepatocytes including the CYP activities have been much lower than those of human hepatocytes. Another problem is that we do not have an appropriate culture system to maintain mature phenotypes of adult hepatocytes. Even if researchers succeed in generating iPS cell-derived hepatocytes with authentically mature phenotypes, it is very likely that their hepatic functions will last only for a short period, a likelihood that this will hamper implementation of drug screening programs that take longer than several weeks. Thus, it is crucial to explore an appropriate culture system for maintaining mature hepatocytes.

5.3. Disease Model

Two major challenges in the application of iPS cell-derived hepatocytes in disease model are the kinetics of disease onset and progression as well as the spatial localization of a disease in the patient's body [8]. First, it may be difficult or not practical to model diseases *in vitro* with a long latency. One possible solution to this challenge would be attempting to accelerate the onset of pathological phenotypes by exposing the cells to environmental effects that may contribute to the disease. In such a strategy, however, researchers have to be careful about the results, since the imposed environment may produce artifacts. Second, it may be difficult or impractical to model hepatic diseases *in vitro* only with hepatocytes. Currently, possible interactions of hepatocytes that are affected in a patient with other cell types within the liver or within the diseased patient's body have not yet been systematically reconstructed.

6. Possibility of Direct Conversion of Somatic Differentiated or Stem Cells into Functional Hepatocytes

The direct conversion of somatic cells into functional hepatocytes may offer a useful technique in cell replacement therapy. Such a strategy might make it possible to circumvent the risks in the therapeutic application of iPS cell-derived hepatocytes, such as the teratoma formation problem. In addition, the omission of the process to reprogram somatic cells to pluripotency would be more convenient.

It has been demonstrated that one type of differentiated cell can be directly converted into another type without requiring a stem-cell intermediate stage. This strategy is conceptually based on that for the generation of iPS cells from differentiated somatic cells. Zhou *et al.* demonstrated that *in vivo* adenoviral expression of key developmental regulators, namely three transcription factors (Ngn3, Pdx1 and Mafa), reprogrammed differentiated pancreatic exocrine cells in adult mice into β-like cells [91]. Feng *et al.* reported retroviral expression of transcription factors PU.1 and C/EBPα converted fibroblasts into macrophage-like cells [92]. More recently, Vierbuchen *et al.* have demonstrated that combinatorial expression of neural-lineage-specific transcription factors via lentiviral vectors directly converted fibroblasts to functional neurons [93]. As described above, ectopic expression of key transcription factors is possible for converting one cell type to another. So far there have been no reports on the direct conversion of differentiated cells into hepatocytes using such methods. That, however, may be changed in the not-too-distant future because several transcription factors have been defined which play a key role in hepatic development: HEX, FOXA1 and FOXA2, GATA4 and GATA6, HNF1α and HNF4, and C/EBPα [94]. Ectopic expression of these transcription factors in a combinatorial and/or sequential manner might be feasible for generating hepatocytes directly from other types of differentiated cells such as fibroblasts.

Another, and probably the best-known candidate for the somatic cell origin for direct conversion into hepatocytes is mesenchymal stem cells (MSCs). MSCs are present in adult mesodermal tissues such as the bone marrow, the adipose tissue and the cartilage, and can differentiate into several types of mesodermal cells – osteoblasts, chondrocytes, adipocytes, and myoblasts – under varying culture conditions [95]. In addition, it has been demonstrated that MSCs have “stem cell plasticity”, the ability of adult stem cells to cross lineage barriers to adopt the expression profile and functional phenotypes of cells unique to other tissues including the liver [96]. Previous studies from our laboratory demonstrated that human adipose tissue-derived MSCs exhibited an *in vitro* hepatic differentiation ability when cultured using a protocol similar to that for directing ES cells into hepatocytes [97,98]. When transplanted into CCl_4-injured mice, the transdifferentiated hepatocytes were incorporated into the host livers. This brought about improvement in some liver functions such as levels of ammnonia concentration and glutamic-pyruvate transaminase. It is of note that transdifferentiation of MSCs into hepatocytes does not involve viral transduction, which offers safety in their use in a clinical application.

Although each strategy described above holds promise for partly circumventing the obstacles confronted by iPS cells, each has challenging issues to overcome prior to clinical application. Since direct conversion of differentiated somatic cells into hepatocytes involves viral transduction, they would share the unpredictable problems with iPS cells as described earlier. MSCs also hold possible risks in therapeutic use. The principal concern in the use of MSCs is the complexity of their interaction with cancer. The effects of MSCs, which secrete a variety of cytokines, on the progression of primary tumors can be pro- as well as anti-tumorigenic [99]. In addition, concerns have been raised about whether MSCs are the putative originating cells of sarcomas, malignant tumors that arise from the mesoderm [100]. Further and thorough investigation regarding these issues is necessary.

Conclusion

The study on techniques to generate iPS cells has undergone tremendous growth over the last several years. Accordingly, evidence has been accumulating that generated iPS cells give rise to a variety of differentiated cell types, including hepatocytes. In concert with this progress are the increasing expectations that iPS cell-derived hepatocytes can serve as an alternative cell source to human hepatocytes in cell replacement therapy, drug screening, and disease model. However, researchers must validate the feasibility of applying these techniques as carefully as possible from the points of view of current challenging issues, including the confirmation of safety, the elucidation of reprogramming mechanisms, and a thorough characterization of iPS cells as well as iPS cell-derived hepatocytes. Concomitantly, researchers must establish ways to evaluate each iPS cell line and stringent criteria for clinical application. As challenging as these issues are, the potential of iPS cell technology is very promising. Considering the current rapid progress in this field, iPS cell technology could ultimately bring innovation to medicine in the not-too-distant future.

References

[1] Dollé L, Best J, Mei J, Al Battah F, Reynaert H, van Grunsven LA, and Geerts A. The quest for liver progenitor cells: a practical point of view. *J Hepatol.* 2010 Jan;52(1):117-29.

[2] Demetriou AA, Brown RS Jr, Busuttil RW, Fair J, McGuire BM, Rosenthal P, Am Esch JS 2nd, Lerut J, Nyberg SL, Salizzoni M, Fagan EA, de Hemptinne B, Broelsch CE, Muraca M, Salmeron JM, Rabkin JM, Metselaar HJ, Pratt D, De La Mata M, McChesney LP, Everson GT, Lavin PT, Stevens AC, Pitkin Z, and Solomon BA. Prospective, randomized, multicenter, controlled trial of a bioartificial liver in treating acute liver failure. *Ann Surg*. 2004 May;239(5):660-7.

[3] Hewitt NJ, Lechón MJ, Houston JB, Hallifax D, Brown HS, Maurel P, Kenna JG, Gustavsson L, Lohmann C, Skonberg C, Guillouzo A, Tuschl G, Li AP, LeCluyse E, Groothuis GM, and Hengstler JG. Primary hepatocytes: current understanding of the regulation of metabolic enzymes and transporter proteins, and pharmaceutical practice for the use of hepatocytes in metabolism, enzyme induction, transporter, clearance, and hepatotoxicity studies. *Drug Metab Rev*. 2007;39(1):159-234.

[4] Azuma H, Paulk N, Ranade A, Dorrell C, Al-Dhalimy M, Ellis E, Strom S, Kay MA, Finegold M, and Grompe M. Robust expansion of human hepatocytes in Fah-/-/Rag2-/-/Il2rg-/- mice. *Nat Biotechnol*. 2007 Aug;25(8):903-10.

[5] Keller GM. *In vitro* differentiation of embryonic stem cells. *Curr Opin Cell Biol*. 1995 Dec;7(6):862-9.

[6] Thomson JA, Itskovitz-Eldor J, Shapiro SS, Waknitz MA, Swiergiel JJ, Marshall VS, and Jones JM. Embryonic stem cell lines derived from human blastocysts. *Science*. 1998 Nov 6;282(5391):1145-7.

[7] Ochiya T, Yamamoto Y, and Banas A. Commitment of stem cells into functional hepatocytes. *Differentiation*. 2010 Feb;79(2):65-73.

[8] Saha K and Jaenisch R. Technical challenges in using human induced pluripotent stem cells to model disease. *Cell Stem Cell.* 2009 Dec 4;5(6):584-95.

[9] Takahashi K and Yamanaka S. Induction of pluripotent stem cells from mouse embryonic and adult fibroblast cultures by defined factors. *Cell.* 2006 Aug 25;126(4):663-76.

[10] Takahashi K, Tanabe K, Ohnuki M, Narita M, Ichisaka T, Tomoda K, and Yamanaka S. Induction of pluripotent stem cells from adult human fibroblasts by defined factors. *Cell.* 2007 Nov 30;131(5):861-72.

[11] Meissner A, Wernig M, and Jaenisch R. Direct reprogramming of genetically unmodified fibroblasts into pluripotent stem cells. *Nat Biotechnol.* 2007 Oct;25(10):1177-81.

[12] Okita K, Ichisaka T, and Yamanaka S. Generation of germline-competent induced pluripotent stem cells. *Nature.* 2007 Jul 19;448(7151):313-7.

[13] Wernig M, Meissner A, Foreman R, Brambrink T, Ku M, Hochedlinger K, Bernstein BE, and Jaenisch R. *In vitro* reprogramming of fibroblasts into a pluripotent ES-cell-like state. *Nature.* 2007 Jul 19;448(7151):318-24.

[14] Park IH, Zhao R, West JA, Yabuuchi A, Huo H, Ince TA, Lerou PH, Lensch MW, and Daley GQ. Reprogramming of human somatic cells to pluripotency with defined factors. *Nature.* 2008 Jan 10;451(7175):141-6.

[15] Yu J, Vodyanik MA, Smuga-Otto K, Antosiewicz-Bourget J, Frane JL, Tian S, Nie J, Jonsdottir GA, Ruotti V, Stewart R, Slukvin II, and Thomson JA. Induced pluripotent stem cell lines derived from human somatic cells. *Science.* 2007 Dec 21;318(5858):1917-20.

[16] Nakagawa M, Koyanagi M, Tanabe K, Takahashi K, Ichisaka T, Aoi T, Okita K, Mochiduki Y, Takizawa N, and Yamanaka S. Generation of induced pluripotent stem cells without Myc from mouse and human fibroblasts. *Nat Biotechnol.* 2008 Jan;26(1):101-6.

[17] Kim JB, Sebastiano V, Wu G, Araúzo-Bravo MJ, Sasse P, Gentile L, Ko K, Ruau D, Ehrich M, van den Boom D, Meyer J, Hübner K, Bernemann C, Ortmeier C, Zenke M, Fleischmann BK, Zaehres H, and Schöler HR. Oct4-induced pluripotency in adult neural stem cells. *Cell.* 2009 Feb 6;136(3):411-9.

[18] Kaji K, Norrby K, Paca A, Mileikovsky M, Mohseni P, and Woltjen K. Virus-free induction of pluripotency and subsequent excision of reprogramming factors. *Nature.* 2009 Apr 9;458(7239):771-5.

[19] Warren L, Manos PD, Ahfeldt T, Loh YH, Li H, Lau F, Ebina W, Mandal PK, Smith ZD, Meissner A, Daley GQ, Brack AS, Collins JJ, Cowan C, Schlaeger TM, and Rossi DJ. Highly efficient reprogramming to pluripotency and directed differentiation of human cells with synthetic modified mRNA. *Cell Stem Cell.* 2010 Nov 5;7(5):618-30.

[20] Soldner F, Hockemeyer D, Beard C, Gao Q, Bell GW, Cook EG, Hargus G, Blak A, Cooper O, Mitalipova M, Isacson O, and Jaenisch R. Parkinson's disease patient-derived induced pluripotent stem cells free of viral reprogramming factors. *Cell.* 2009 Mar 6;136(5):964-77.

[21] Woltjen K, Michael IP, Mohseni P, Desai R, Mileikovsky M, Hämäläinen R, Cowling R, Wang W, Liu P, Gertsenstein M, Kaji K, Sung HK, and Nagy A. piggyBac transposition reprograms fibroblasts to induced pluripotent stem cells. *Nature.* 2009 Apr 9;458(7239):766-70.

[22] Huangfu D, Osafune K, Maehr R, Guo W, Eijkelenboom A, Chen S, Muhlestein W, and Melton DA. Induction of pluripotent stem cells from primary human fibroblasts with only Oct4 and Sox2. *Nat Biotechnol.* 2008 Nov;26(11):1269-75.

[23] Zhou H, Wu S, Joo JY, Zhu S, Han DW, Lin T, Trauger S, Bien G, Yao S, Zhu Y, Siuzdak G, Schöler HR, Duan L, and Ding S. Generation of induced pluripotent stem cells using recombinant proteins. *Cell Stem Cell.* 2009 May 8;4(5):381-4.

[24] Tian T and Meng AM. Nodal signals pattern vertebrate embryos. *Cell Mol Life Sci.* 2006 Mar;63(6):672-85.

[25] Lowe LA, Yamada S, and Kuehn MR. Genetic dissection of nodal function in patterning the mouse embryo. *Development.* 2001 May;128(10):1831-43.

[26] Vincent SD, Dunn NR, Hayashi S, Norris DP, and Robertson EJ. Cell fate decisions within the mouse organizer are governed by graded Nodal signals. *Genes Dev.* 2003 Jul 1;17(13):1646-62.

[27] Bossard P, and Zaret KS. GATA transcription factors as potentiators of gut endoderm differentiation. *Development.* 1998 Dec;125(24):4909-17.

[28] Cirillo LA, Lin FR, Cuesta I, Friedman D, Jarnik M, and Zaret KS. Opening of compacted chromatin by early developmental transcription factors HNF3 (FoxA) and GATA-4. *Mol Cell.* 2002 Feb;9(2):279-89.

[29] Jung J, Zheng M, Goldfarb M, and Zaret KS. Initiation of mammalian liver development from endoderm by fibroblast growth factors. *Science.* 1999 Jun 18;284(5422):1998-2003.

[30] Rossi JM, Dunn NR, Hogan BL, and Zaret KS. Distinct mesodermal signals, including BMPs from the septum transversum mesenchyme, are

required in combination for hepatogenesis from the endoderm. *Genes Dev.* 2001 Aug 1;15(15):1998-2009.

[31] Bort R, Signore M, Tremblay K, Martinez Barbera JP, and Zaret KS. Hex homeobox gene controls the transition of the endoderm to a pseudostratified, cell emergent epithelium for liver bud development. *Dev Biol.* 2006 Feb 1;290(1):44-56.

[32] Sosa-Pineda B, Wigle JT, and Oliver G. Hepatocyte migration during liver development requires Prox1. *Nat Genet.* 2000 Jul;25(3):254-5.

[33] Schmidt C, Bladt F, Goedecke S, Brinkmann V, Zschiesche W, Sharpe M, Gherardi E, and Birchmeier C. Scatter factor/hepatocyte growth factor is essential for liver development. *Nature.* 1995 Feb 23;373(6516):699-702.

[34] Ishikawa KS, Masui T, Ishikawa K, and Shiojiri N. Immunolocalization of hepatocyte growth factor and its receptor (c-Met) during mouse liver development. *Histochem Cell Biol.* 2001 Nov;116(5):453-62.

[35] Kamiya A, Kinoshita T, Ito Y, Matsui T, Morikawa Y, Senba E, Nakashima K, Taga T, Yoshida K, Kishimoto T, and Miyajima. Fetal liver development requires a paracrine action of oncostatin M through the gp130 signal transducer. *EMBO J.* 1999 Apr 15;18(8):2127-36.

[36] Kamiya A, Kinoshita T, and Miyajima A. Oncostatin M and hepatocyte growth factor induce hepatic maturation via distinct signaling pathways. *FEBS Lett.* 2001 Mar 9;492(1-2):90-4.

[37] Hamazaki T, Iiboshi Y, Oka M, Papst PJ, Meacham AM, Zon LI, and Terada N. Hepatic maturation in differentiating embryonic stem cells *in vitro*. *FEBS Lett.* 2001 May 18;497(1):15-9.

[38] Chinzei R, Tanaka Y, Shimizu-Saito K, Hara Y, Kakinuma S, Watanabe M, Teramoto K, Arii S, Takase K, Sato C, Terada N, and Teraoka H. Embryoid-body cells derived from a mouse embryonic stem cell line show differentiation into functional hepatocytes. *Hepatology.* 2002 Jul;36(1):22-9.

[39] Jones EA, Tosh D, Wilson DI, Lindsay S, and Forrester LM. Hepatic differentiation of murine embryonic stem cells. *Exp Cell Res.* 2002 Jan 1;272(1):15-22.

[40] Yamada T, Yoshikawa M, Kanda S, Kato Y, Nakajima Y, Ishizaka S, and Tsunoda Y. *In vitro* differentiation of embryonic stem cells into hepatocyte-like cells identified by cellular uptake of indocyanine green. *Stem Cells.* 2002;20(2):146-54.

[41] Miyashita H, Suzuki A, Fukao K, Nakauchi H, and Taniguchi H. Evidence for hepatocyte differentiation from embryonic stem cells *in vitro*. *Cell Transplant.* 2002;11(5):429-34.

[42] Kuai XL, Cong XQ, Li XL, and Xiao SD. Generation of hepatocytes from cultured mouse embryonic stem cells. *Liver Transpl.* 2003 Oct;9(10):1094-9.

[43] Gouon-Evans V, Boussemart L, Gadue P, Nierhoff D, Koehler CI, Kubo A, Shafritz DA, and Keller G. BMP-4 is required for hepatic specification of mouse embryonic stem cell-derived definitive endoderm. *Nat Biotechnol.* 2006 Nov;24(11):1402-11.

[44] Soto-Gutiérrez A, Navarro-Alvarez N, Zhao D, Rivas-Carrillo JD, Lebkowski J, Tanaka N, Fox IJ, and Kobayashi N. Differentiation of mouse embryonic stem cells to hepatocyte-like cells by co-culture with human liver nonparenchymal cell lines. *Nat Protoc.* 2007;2(2):347-56.

[45] Teratani T, Yamamoto H, Aoyagi K, Sasaki H, Asari A, Quinn G, Sasaki H, Terada M, and Ochiya T. Direct hepatic fate specification from mouse embryonic stem cells. *Hepatology.* 2005 Apr;41(4):836-46.

[46] Cai J, Zhao Y, Liu Y, Ye F, Song Z, Qin H, Meng S, Chen Y, Zhou R, Song X, Guo Y, Ding M, and Deng H. Directed differentiation of human embryonic stem cells into functional hepatic cells. *Hepatology.* 2007 May;45(5):1229-39.

[47] Hay DC, Zhao D, Ross A, Mandalam R, Lebkowski J, and Cui W. Direct differentiation of human embryonic stem cells to hepatocyte-like cells exhibiting functional activities. *Cloning Stem Cells.* 2007 Spring;9(1):51-62.

[48] Hay DC, Zhao D, Fletcher J, Hewitt ZA, McLean D, Urruticoechea-Uriguen A, Black JR, Elcombe C, Ross JA, Wolf R, and Cui W. Efficient differentiation of hepatocytes from human embryonic stem cells exhibiting markers recapitulating liver development *in vivo*. *Stem Cells.* 2008 Apr;26(4):894-902.

[49] de Caestecker M. The transforming growth factor-beta superfamily of receptors. Cytokine Growth Factor Rev. 2004 Feb;15(1):1-11.

[50] D'Amour KA, Agulnick AD, Eliazer S, Kelly OG, Kroon E, and Baetge EE. Efficient differentiation of human embryonic stem cells to definitive endoderm. *Nat Biotechnol.* 2005 Dec;23(12):1534-41.

[51] Mizejewski GJ. Alpha-fetoprotein structure and function: relevance to isoforms, epitopes, and conformational variants. *Exp Biol Med* (Maywood). 2001 May;226(5):377-408.

[52] Song Z, Cai J, Liu Y, Zhao D, Yong J, Duo S, Song X, Guo Y, Zhao Y, Qin H, Yin X, Wu C, Che J, Lu S, Ding M, and Deng H. Efficient generation of hepatocyte-like cells from human induced pluripotent stem cells. *Cell Res.* 2009 Nov;19(11):1233-42.

[53] Si-Tayeb K, Noto FK, Nagaoka M, Li J, Battle MA, Duris C, North PE, Dalton S, and Duncan SA. Highly efficient generation of human hepatocyte-like cells from induced pluripotent stem cells. *Hepatology.* 2010 Jan;51(1):297-305.

[54] Sullivan GJ, Hay DC, Park IH, Fletcher J, Hannoun Z, Payne CM, Dalgetty D, Black JR, Ross JA, Samuel K, Wang G, Daley GQ, Lee JH, Church GM, Forbes SJ, Iredale JP, and Wilmut I. Generation of functional human hepatic endoderm from human induced pluripotent stem cells. *Hepatology.* 2010 Jan;51(1):329-35.

[55] Li W, Wang D, Qin J, Liu C, Zhang Q, Zhang X, Yu X, Lahn BT, Mao FF, and Xiang AP. Generation of functional hepatocytes from mouse induced pluripotent stem cells. *J Cell Physiol.* 2010 Mar;222(3):492-501.

[56] Gai H, Nguyen DM, Moon YJ, Aguila JR, Fink LM, Ward DC, and Ma Y. Generation of murine hepatic lineage cells from induced pluripotent stem cells. *Differentiation.* 2010 Mar;79(3):171-81.

[57] Liu H, Ye Z, Kim Y, Sharkis S, and Jang YY. Generation of endoderm-derived human induced pluripotent stem cells from primary hepatocytes. *Hepatology.* 2010 May;51(5):1810-9.

[58] Touboul T, Hannan NR, Corbineau S, Martinez A, Martinet C, Branchereau S, Mainot S, Strick-Marchand H, Pedersen R, Di Santo J, Weber A, and Vallier L. Generation of functional hepatocytes from human embryonic stem cells under chemically defined conditions that recapitulate liver development. *Hepatology.* 2010 May;51(5):1754-65.

[59] Espejel S, Roll GR, McLaughlin KJ, Lee AY, Zhang JY, Laird DJ, Okita K, Yamanaka S, and Willenbring H. Induced pluripotent stem cell-derived hepatocytes have the functional and proliferative capabilities needed for liver regeneration in mice. *J Clin Invest.* 2010 Sep 1;120(9):3120-6.

[60] Rashid ST, Corbineau S, Hannan N, Marciniak SJ, Miranda E, Alexander G, Huang-Doran I, Griffin J, Ahrlund-Richter L, Skepper J, Semple R, Weber A, Lomas DA, and Vallier L. Modeling inherited metabolic disorders of the liver using human induced pluripotent stem cells. *J Clin Invest.* 2010 Sep 1;120(9):3127-36.

[61] Huang HP, Yu CY, Chen HF, Chen PH, Chuang CY, Lin SJ, Huang ST, Chan WH, Ueng TH, Ho HN, and Kuo HC. Factors from human embryonic stem cell-derived fibroblast-like cells promote topology-dependent hepatic differentiation in primate embryonic and induced pluripotent stem cells. *J Biol Chem*. 2010 Oct 22;285(43):33510-9.

[62] Ghodsizadeh A, Taei A, Totonchi M, Seifinejad A, Gourabi H, Pournasr B, Aghdami N, Malekzadeh R, Almadani N, Salekdeh GH, and Baharvand H. Generation of liver disease-specific induced pluripotent stem cells along with efficient differentiation to functional hepatocyte-like cells. *Stem Cell Rev*. 2010 Dec;6(4):622-32.

[63] Inamura M, Kawabata K, Takayama K, Tashiro K, Sakurai F, Katayama K, Toyoda M, Akutsu H, Miyagawa Y, Okita H, Kiyokawa N, Umezawa A, Hayakawa T, Furue MK, and Mizuguchi H. Efficient generation of hepatoblasts from human ES cells and iPS cells by transient overexpression of homeobox gene HEX. *Mol Ther*. 2011 Feb;19(2):400-7.

[64] Iwamuro M, Komaki T, Kubota Y, Seita M, Kawamoto H, Yuasa T, Shahid JM, Hassan RA, Hassan WA, Nakaji S, Nishikawa Y, Kondo E, Yamamoto K, Fox IJ, and Kobayashi N. Hepatic differentiation of mouse iPS cells *in vitro*. *Cell Transplant*. 2010;19(6):841-7.

[65] Sancho-Bru P, Roelandt P, Narain N, Pauwelyn K, Notelaers T, Shimizu T, Ott M, and Verfaillie C. Directed differentiation of murine-induced pluripotent stem cells to functional hepatocyte-like cells. *J Hepatol*. 2011 Jan;54(1):98-107.

[66] Jozefczuk J, Prigione A, Chavez L, and Adjaye J. Comparative analysis of human embryonic stem cell and induced pluripotent stem cell-derived hepatocyte-like cells reveals current drawbacks and possible strategies for improved differentiation. Stem *Cells Dev*. 2011 Jan 24. [Epub ahead of print]

[67] Ohashi K. Liver tissue engineering: The future of liver therapeutics. *Hepatol Res*. 2008 Nov;38(Suppl.1):S76-S87.

[68] Sakai Y, Huang H, Hanada S, and Niino T. Toward engineering of vascularized three-dimensional liver tissue equivalents possessing a clinically significant mass. *Biochem Eng J*. 2010 Feb;48(3):348-361.

[69] Hanna J, Wernig M, Markoulaki S, Sun CW, Meissner A, Cassady JP, Beard C, Brambrink T, Wu LC, Townes TM, and Jaenisch R. Treatment of sickle cell anemia mouse model with iPS cells generated from autologous skin. *Science*. 2007 Dec 21;318(5858):1920-3.

[70] Raya A, Rodríguez-Pizà I, Guenechea G, Vassena R, Navarro S, Barrero MJ, Consiglio A, Castellà M, Río P, Sleep E, González F, Tiscornia G, Garreta E, Aasen T, Veiga A, Verma IM, Surrallés J, Bueren J, and Izpisúa Belmonte JC. Disease-corrected haematopoietic progenitors from Fanconi anaemia induced pluripotent stem cells. *Nature*. 2009 Jul 2;460(7251):53-9.

[71] Kazuki Y, Hiratsuka M, Takiguchi M, Osaki M, Kajitani N, Hoshiya H, Hiramatsu K, Yoshino T, Kazuki K, Ishihara C, Takehara S, Higaki K, Nakagawa M, Takahashi K, Yamanaka S, and Oshimura M. Complete genetic correction of iPS cells from Duchenne muscular dystrophy. *Mol Ther*. 2010 Feb;18(2):386-93.

[72] Kobayashi T, Yamaguchi T, Hamanaka S, Kato-Itoh M, Yamazaki Y, Ibata M, Sato H, Lee YS, Usui J, Knisely AS, Hirabayashi M, and Nakauchi H. Generation of rat pancreas in mouse by interspecific blastocyst injection of pluripotent stem cells. *Cell*. 2010 Sep 3;142(5):787-99.

[73] Guengerich FP. Cytochrome p450 and chemical toxicology. *Chem Res Toxicol*. 2008 Jan;21(1):70-83.

[74] Rebouissou S, Amessou M, Couchy G, Poussin K, Imbeaud S, Pilati C, Izard T, Balabaud C, Bioulac-Sage P, and Zucman-Rossi J. Frequent in-frame somatic deletions activate gp130 in inflammatory hepatocellular tumours. *Nature*. 2009 Jan 8;457(7226):200-4.

[75] Laurent-Puig P and Zucman-Rossi J. Genetics of hepatocellular tumors. *Oncogene*. 2006 Jun 26;25(27):3778-86.

[76] Bluteau O, Jeannot E, Bioulac-Sage P, Marqués JM, Blanc JF, Bui H, Beaudoin JC, Franco D, Balabaud C, Laurent-Puig P, and Zucman-Rossi J. Bi-allelic inactivation of TCF1 in hepatic adenomas. *Nat Genet*. 2002 Oct;32(2):312-5.

[77] Wong CM, Fan ST, and Ng IO. β-Catenin mutation and overexpression in hepatocellular carcinoma: clinicopathologic and prognostic significance. *Cancer*. 2001 Jul 1;92(1):136-45.

[78] Tanaka S, Toh Y, Adachi E, Matsumata T, Mori R, and Sugimachi K. Tumor progression in hepatocellular carcinoma may be mediated by p53 mutation. *Cancer Res*. 1993 Jun 15;53(12):2884-7.

[79] Lowry WE, Richter L, Yachechko R, Pyle AD, Tchieu J, Sridharan R, Clark AT, and Plath K. Generation of human induced pluripotent stem cells from dermal fibroblasts. *Proc Natl Acad Sci U S A*. 2008 Feb 26;105(8):2883-8.

[80] Ye Z, Zhan H, Mali P, Dowey S, Williams DM, Jang YY, Dang CV, Spivak JL, Moliterno AR, and Cheng L. Human-induced pluripotent stem cells from blood cells of healthy donors and patients with acquired blood disorders. *Blood.* 2009 Dec 24;114(27):5473-80.

[81] Kim JB, Greber B, Araúzo-Bravo MJ, Meyer J, Park KI, Zaehres H, and Schöler HR. Direct reprogramming of human neural stem cells by OCT4. *Nature*. 2009 Oct 1;461(7264):649-3.

[82] Aasen T, Raya A, Barrero MJ, Garreta E, Consiglio A, Gonzalez F, Vassena R, Bilić J, Pekarik V, Tiscornia G, Edel M, Boué S, Izpisúa, and Belmonte JC. Efficient and rapid generation of induced pluripotent stem cells from human keratinocytes. *Nat Biotechnol.* 2008 Nov;26(11):1276-84.

[83] Gutierrez-Aranda I, Ramos-Mejia V, Bueno C, Munoz-Lopez M, Real PJ, Mácia A, Sanchez L, Ligero G, Garcia-Parez JL, and Menendez P. Human induced pluripotent stem cells develop teratoma more efficiently and faster than human embryonic stem cells regardless the site of injection. *Stem Cells*. 2010 Sep;28(9):1568-70.

[84] Yamanaka S. A fresh look at iPS cells. *Cell.* 2009 Apr 3;137(1):13-7.

[85] Fairchild PJ. The challenge of immunogenicity in the quest for induced pluripotency. *Nat Rev Immunol.* 2010 Dec;10(12):868-75.

[86] Chin MH, Mason MJ, Xie W, Volinia S, Singer M, Peterson C, Ambartsumyan G, Aimiuwu O, Richter L, Zhang J, Khvorostov I, Ott V, Grunstein M, Lavon N, Benvenisty N, Croce CM, Clark AT, Baxter T, Pyle AD, Teitell MA, Pelegrini M, Plath K, and Lowry WE. Induced pluripotent stem cells and embryonic stem cells are distinguished by gene expression signatures. *Cell Stem Cell.* 2009 Jul 2;5(1):111-23.

[87] Neveu P, Kye MJ, Qi S, Buchholz DE, Clegg DO, Sahin M, Park IH, Kim KS, Daley GQ, Kornblum HI, Shraiman BI, and Kosik KS. MicroRNA profiling reveals two distinct p53-related human pluripotent stem cell states. *Cell Stem Cell.* 2010 Dec 3;7(6):671-81.

[88] Doi A, Park IH, Wen B, Murakami P, Aryee MJ, Irizarry R, Herb B, Ladd-Acosta C, Rho J, Loewer S, Miller J, Schlaeger T, Daley GQ, and Feinberg AP. Differential methylation of tissue- and cancer-specific CpG island shores distinguishes human induced pluripotent stem cells, embryonic stem cells and fibroblasts. *Nat Genet.* 2009 Dec;41(12):1350-3.

[89] Pick M, Stelzer Y, Bar-Nur O, Mayshar Y, Eden A, and Benvenisty N. Clone- and gene-specific aberrations of parental imprinting in human induced pluripotent stem cells. *Stem Cells*. 2009 Nov;27(11):2686-90.

[90] Miura K, Okada Y, Aoi T, Okada A, Takahashi K, Okita K, Nakagawa M, Koyanagi M, Tanabe K, Ohnuki M, Ogawa D, Ikeda E, Okano H, and Yamanaka S. Variation in the safety of induced pluripotent stem cell lines. *Nat Biotechnol.* 2009 Aug;27(8):743-5.

[91] Zhou Q, Brown J, Kanarek A, Rajagopal J, and Melton DA. *In vivo* reprogramming of adult pancreatic exocrine cells to beta-cells. *Nature.* 2008 Oct 2;455(7213):627-32.

[92] Feng R, Desbordes SC, Xie H, Tillo ES, Pixley F, Stanley ER, and Graf T. PU.1 and C/EBPα/β convert fibroblasts into macrophage-like cells. *Proc Natl Acad Sci U S A.* 2008 Apr 22;105(16):6057-62.

[93] Vierbuchen T, Ostermeier A, Pang ZP, Kokubu Y, Südhof TC, and Wernig M. Direct conversion of fibroblasts to functional neurons by defined factors. *Nature.* 2010 Feb 25;463(7284):1035-41.

[94] Tanimizu N and Miyajima A. Molecular mechanism of liver development and regeneration. *Int Rev Cytol.* 2007;259:1-48.

[95] Chamberlain G, Fox J, Ashton B, and Middleton J. Concise review: mesenchymal stem cells: their phenotype, differentiation capacity, immunological features, and potential for homing. *Stem Cells.* 2007 Nov;25(11):2739-49.

[96] Banas A, Yamamoto Y, Teratani T, and Ochiya T. Stem cell plasticity: learning from hepatogenic differentiation strategies. *Dev Dyn.* 2007 Dec;236(12):3228-41.

[97] Banas A, Teratani T, Yamamoto Y, Tokuhara M, Takeshita F, Quinn G, Okochi H, and Ochiya T. Adipose tissue-derived mesenchymal stem cells as a source of human hepatocytes. *Hepatology.* 2007 Jul;46(1):219-28.

[98] Banas A, Teratani T, Yamamoto Y, Tokuhara M, Takeshita F, Osaki M, Kato T, Okochi H, and Ochiya T. Rapid hepatic fate specification of adipose-derived stem cells and their therapeutic potential for liver failure. *J Gastroenterol Hepatol.* 2009 Jan;24(1):70-7.

[99] Bergfeld SA and Declerck YA. Bone marrow-derived mesenchymal stem cells and the tumor microenvironment. *Cancer Metastasis Rev.* 2010 Jun;29(2):249-61.

[100] Mohseny AB and Hogendoorn PC. Mesenchymal tumors: when stem cells go mad. *Stem Cells.* 2011 Jan 7. [Epub ahead of print].

In: Induced Stem Cells
Editors: P. Sullivan and E. Mortensen
ISBN: 978-1-61324-613-9

Chapter IV

Production of Cells with the Patient's Genotype by Induced Pluripotent Stem Cell Technique

Stina Simonsson, Dzeneta Vizlin-Hodzic, Lars Enochson, Cecilia Borestrom and Anders Lindahl
Gothenburg University; Gothenburg, Sweden

In 2006, it was reported that only four transcription factors were needed to remarkably reprogram mouse fibroblasts into cells similar to embryonic stem cells (ESCs) and those reprogrammed cells were named induced pluripotent stem cells (iPSCs). The year after, human iPSCs were produced and in 2008 reprogramming cells was chosen as the breakthrough of the year by Science magazine. In particular, this was due to the establishment of patient-specific cell lines from patients with various diseases using the induced pluripotent stem cell (iPSC) technique and also due to exciting scientific reports of direct reprogramming of somatic cells into other cell types, not necessary via a pluripotent cell state. The iPSCs can be generated by insertion of genes that turn back the developmental status of cells. These cells can be patient specific and therefore may prove useful in screens for potential drugs, regenerative medicine, increasing knowledge of human development, and in models for specific human diseases. This chapter provides a summary of cell types of human origin that have been transformed into iPSCs and of different iPSC procedures that exist. Further we discuss advantages and disadvantages of procedures, potential medical applications and implications that may arise in the iPSC field due to the resent report that reprogramming occurs using only retrovirus excluding transgenic transcription factors.

Preface

The differentiated state of adult somatic cells has been considered very stable, but has experimentally been shown to be reversible. The ultimate proof is cloning animals, resulting in a new individual from one differentiated somatic cell. Reprogramming has experimentally been achieved by 1) somatic cell nuclear transfer (SCNT) to eggs (cloning), 2) cell fusion, 3) exposure in egg extract and 4) overexpression of transcription factors to generate induced pluripotent stem cells (iPSCs). The mechanisms of nuclear reprogramming are not yet completely understood and several ways of generating iPSCs exist and entails 1) overexpression of different combinations of transcription factors most efficiently in combination with retroviruses, 2) exposure to chemical compounds in combination with the transcription factors Oct4, Klf4 and retroviruses, or 3) retroviruses alone. The resulting reprogrammed cells are in a naïve pluripotent cell state and can from there be redirected into most if not all different differentiation pathways probably depending on the grade of reprogramming and the pluripotent state. Generation of patient-specific iPSC lines capable of giving rise to any desired cell type provides great opportunities to treat many disorders either as transplantation of healthy cells/tissue (Route 1 in Figure 1) or discovery of patient specific medicines in human iPSC model system (Route 2 in Figure 1).Here, some of this field's fast progress and results mostly concerning human cells are summarized.

Induced Pluripotent Stem Cells (iPSCs)

In 2006, a brilliant report was published by Takahashi and Yamanaka (Takahashi and Yamanaka, 2006), showing that only four transcription factors, namely Oct4, Sox2, Klf4 and C-Myc, could be used to reprogram mouse fibroblasts into cells that resemble embryonic stem cells (ESCs) in terms of their morphology, growth rate, cell-surface markers, telomerase activity and differentiation into derivatives of all three embryonic germ layers. These cells were called iPSCs. Takahashi and Yamanaka came up with those four reprogramming proteins after a search for regulators of pluripotency among 24 cherry picked pluripotency-associated genes. These initial iPSC lines differed from ESCs in that they had a diverse global gene expression pattern compared to ESCs and failed to produce adult chimeric mice. Later iPSCs were shown to have the ability to form live chimeric mice and were transmitted through the germ line to offspring when using Oct4 or Nanog as selection marker for reprogramming instead of Fbx15, which was used in the initial experiments (Meissner et al., 2007; Okita et al., 2007; Wernig et al., 2007). In 2007, the first human iPSC lines were successfully generated by Oct4 and Sox2 combined with either, Klf4 and c-Myc, as used earlier in the mouse model, or Nanog and Lin28 (Lowry et al., 2008; Nakagawa et al., 2008; Park et al., 2008b; Takahashi et al., 2007; Yu et al., 2007). Today many laboratories and hospitals worldwide are producing iPSC lines from patients with various diseases. Patient-specific iPSC lines can be used as 1) a human modelling system for studying the molecular cause of, and in the long run for 2) the treatment of, degenerative diseases with autologous transplantation, which refers to the transplantation to a patient of his/her own cells. The therapeutic potential of iPSCs in combination with genetic repair has already been successfully shown in mouse models of sickle cell anemia (Hanna et al., 2007), Duchenne muscular dystrophy (DMD) (Kazuki et al., 2010), hemophilia A (Xu et al., 2009) and, in a rat model, Parkinson's disease (Wernig et al., 2008c). For diseases where animal and human physiology differ, disease-specific iPSC lines capable of differentiation into the tissue affected by the disease could recapitulate tissue formation and thereby enable determination of the cause of the disease and could provide cues to drug targets. Therefore iPSC lines from patients suffering from a variety of genetic diseases with either Mendelian or complex inheritance have been secured for future research, and include deaminase deficiency-related severe combined immunodeficiency (ADA-SCID), Shwachman-Bodian-Diamond syndrome (SBDS), Gaucher disease (GD) type III, Duchenne (DMD) and Becker muscular dystrophy (BMD), Parkinson disease (PD), Huntington disease (HD), juvenile-onset (type1) diabetes mellitus (JDM), Downs syndrome (DS)/trisomy21 and Lesch-Nyhan syndrome (Park et al., 2008a). Furthermore, iPSCs derived from amyotrophic lateral sclerosis (ALS) patients were terminally differentiated into motor neurons (Dimos et al., 2008). The most studied somatic cell type that has been reprogrammed into iPSCs is fibroblasts. The different human somatic cell types that have been transformed into iPSCs so far are summarized in table 1. The efficiency of fibroblast reprogramming does not exceed 1-5% but generally is extremely inefficient (0.001-0.1%) and occurs at a slow speed (> 2 weeks). In order to use iPSCs in clinical applications, improved efficiency, suitable factor delivery techniques and identification of true reprogrammed cells are crucial.

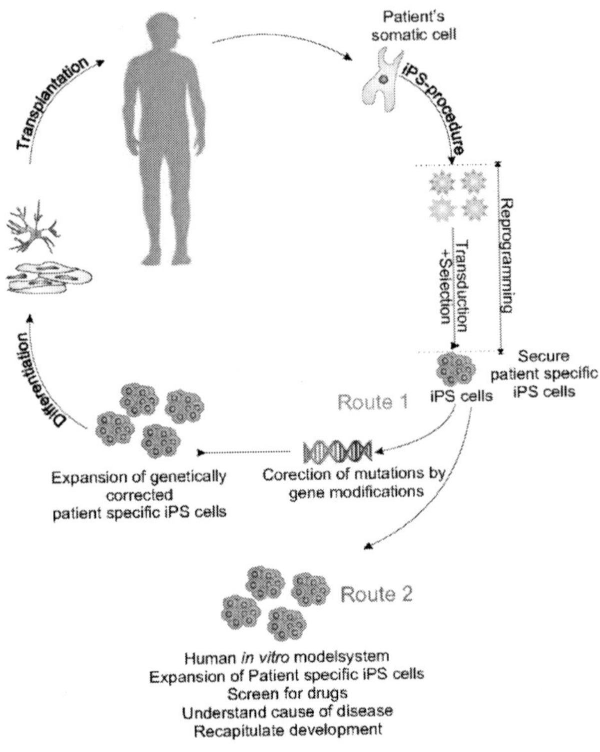

Figure 1. Schematic picture of establishment of patient-specific induced pluripotent stem cell (iPSC) lines, from which two attractive prospective routes emerge i.e. Route 1) *in vivo* transplantation Route 2) *in vitro* applications. Patient-specific embryonic stem (ES)-like cells are produced by collecting adult somatic cells from the patient, for example skin fibroblasts, and in those somatic cells retroviral transduction of defined transcription factors (Oct4 and Sox2 in combination with c-Myc and Klf4 or Lin-28 and Nanog). Reprogrammed iPSCs are selected by the detection of endogenous expression of a reprogramming marker, for example Oct4. First prospective route (Route 1); Generated patient-specific iPSCs can be genetically corrected and upon external signals theoretically stimulated to differentiate into any cell type in the body. In this way, patient-specific dopamine producing nerve cells or skin cells can be generated and transplanted to individuals suffering from Parkinson's disease or Melanoma respectively. Second prospective route (Route 2); Generated disease-specific iPSCs can be used as a human in vitro system to study degenerative disorders, cause of disease and screening for drugs.

Table 1. Different somatic cell types that human iPSCs have been generated from

Human Origin Somatic Cell type	Efficiency	Reprogramming Factors	Reference
Fibroblasts	0.02% 0.02% 0.002%	OKSM OSLN OKS	(Takahashi et al., 2007) (Yu et al., 2007) (Nakagawa et al., 2008)
Hepatocytes	0.1%	OKSM	(Liu et al., 2010)
Keratinocytes	ND ND	OKSM OKS	(Aasen et al., 2008) (Aasen et al., 2008)
Neural stem cells	<0.004%	O	(Kim et al., 2008)
Amniotic cells	0.05-1.5% 0.1%	OKSM OSN	(Li et al., 2009) (Zhao et al., 2010)
Adipose-derived stem cells	0.5% <0.1%	OKSM OKS	(Sugii et al., 2010) (Aoki et al., 2010)
Cord blood stem cells	ND <0.01%	OKSM OS	(Eminli et al., 2009) (Giorgetti et al., 2009)
Cord blood endothelial cells	<0.01%	OSLN	(Haase et al., 2009)
Mobilized peripheral blood	0.01%	OKSM	(Loh et al., 2009)

In the first iPSC reprogramming studies, retroviral or lentiviral vectors were used to introduce the transcription factors into somatic cells. By using these viral delivery systems, the transduced viral vectors and transgenes are randomly and permanently integrated into the genome of infected somatic cells and transmitted to iPSCs. The vector integration into the host genome is a limitation of this technology if it is going to be used in human therapeutic applications due to increased risk of tumor formation (Okita et al., 2007). Approaches to derive transgene-free iPSCs are therefore critically important. The first strategy was by using non-integrating (Figure 2) vectors. Efforts have been made to derive iPSCs by repeated plasmid transfections (Gonzalez et al., 2009; Okita et al., 2008) (Figure 2a), adenoviral (Stadtfeld et al., 2008b) (Figure 2b) and episomal vectors (Yu et al., 2009) (Figure 2c). Recently, minicircle vectors (Figure 2d) have been used to generate iPSCs (Jia et al., 2010). Unfortunately, reprogramming with these techniques has extremely low efficiency as compared to integrating viral vectors. Another promising alternative is the use of excisable integrating vectors, allowing for the generation of transgene-free iPSCs. A classical expression-excision system

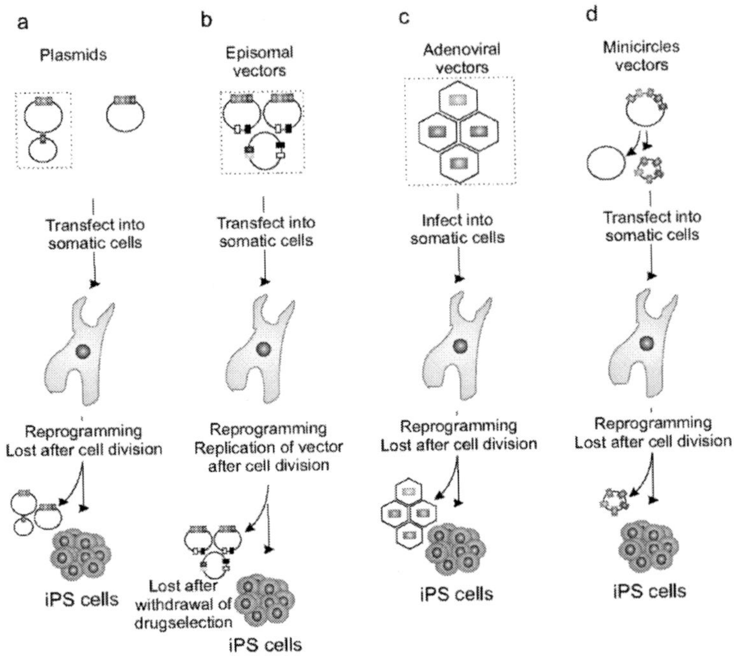

Figure 2. Methods for producing induced pluripotent stem cells (iPSCs) by non-integrating vectors. Several different methods exist to generate iPSCs by non-integrating vectors: for example by plasmid, episomal, adenoviral and minicircle vectors. a) A combination of expression plasmid vectors for defined reprogramming factors is transfected into somatic cells. Plasmid vectors are not integrated into the genome of transfected cells and are gradually lost during reprogramming. This method therefore requires multiple transfection steps. b) Somatic cells can be transfected by episomal vectors expressing defined reprogramming factors. These vectors can replicate themselves autonomously in cells during reprogramming under drug selection and are not integrated into the genome. Upon withdrawal of drug selection, the episomal vectors are lost. c) Adenovirus carrying defined reprogramming factors can be infected into somatic cells to transiently express these factors. This method requires multiple transductions since adenoviral vectors are lost upon celldivision. d) The minicircle vector method is based on PhiC31-vector intra molecular recombinant system that allows the bacterial elements of the vector to be degraded in bacteria. Minicircle vector containing only defined reprogramming factors is not degraded and is delivered into somatic cells by nucleofection. This strategy requires multiple transfection steps since minicircle vectors are lost upon cell division.

uses vectors flanked with recognition sites, loxP sites, for Crerecombinase (Figure 3a). Consequently, DNA is excised upon Cre-recombinase expression in the cells. Cre-loxP-based approaches have been used to reprogram human somatic cells from individuals with Parkinson's disease by four different vectors (Soldner et al., 2009) or by a single, polycistronic lentiviral vector encoding reprogramming factors (Chang et al., 2009). Though, a potential limitation of Cre-loxP-based approaches is that a long terminal repeat (LTR) will remain after Cre-mediated excision which may interfere with the expression of endogenous genes. An alternative integration-free strategy is based on the piggy-Bac transposon (Figure 3b), a mobile genetic element from insects that integrates into the genome of mammalian cells and, most importantly, can be entirely removed by a transposase. Two research teams generated iPSCs using this system to deliver a single polycistron encoding four reprogramming factors into somatic cells (Woltjen et al., 2009; Yusa et al., 2009). Interestingly, the latest development indicates that gene transfection may not even be needed for the generation of iPSCs and that direct delivery of four recombinant reprogramming proteins that can penetrate the plasma membrane of somatic cells is sufficient (Zhou et al., 2009).

The therapeutic application of iPSCs is limited by another concern due to the use of potential oncogenes when iPSCs are produced. C-Myc is an oncogene and as such causes tumor formation, which has been observed in iPSC-derived chimeric mice (Okita et al., 2007). As a major step towards solving this issue, several studies have demonstrated that mouse and human iPSCs can be derived without C-Myc but the efficiency of reprogramming is reduced (Nakagawa et al., 2008; Wernig et al., 2008b; Yu et al., 2007). Although the oncogenic potential of C-Myc is mostly discussed, Oct4, Sox2 and Klf4 are also associated with multiple types of cancer (Bass et al., 2009; Gidekel et al., 2003; Wei et al., 2006). To circumvent this problem, a recent trend is to avoid the transduction of some of the oncogenes by 1) reprogramming somatic cells which already endogenously express sufficient levels of some of the reprogramming factors (Tsai et al., 2010), 2) replacing one or more reprogramming factors by small molecules like histone deacetylase inhibitor vaporic acid, the DNA methyltransferase inhibitor 5-aza-cytidine, the Wnt signaling component WNT3a, the L-channel calcium channel agonist Bayk8644 (Huangfu et al., 2008a; Huangfu et al., 2008b), or 3) dual inhibition of mitogen activated protein kinase signaling and glycogen synthase kinase-3 (Silva et al., 2008). It has been reported that Sox2 can be replaced by Sox1, Klf4 by Klf2 and c-Myc by N-myc or L-myc indicating that they are not fundamentally required for generation of iPSCs (Yamanaka, 2009). Oct4 has not yet been successfully replaced by another member of the Oct family to generate iPSCs and keeping in mind the necessity of Oct4 in early development; Oct4 is the most important factor for reprogramming. However, Blx-01294 an inhibitor of G9a histone methyl transferase, enables neural progenitor cells to be reprogrammed without exogenous Oct4, although transduction of Klf4, c-Myc and Sox2 together with endogenous Oct4 was required (Shi et al., 2008). Recently, Oct4 has been replaced with steroidogenic factor 1, which control Oct4 expression in ESCs by binding the Oct4 proximal promoter, and iPSCs were produced without exogenous Oct4 (Heng et al., 2010).

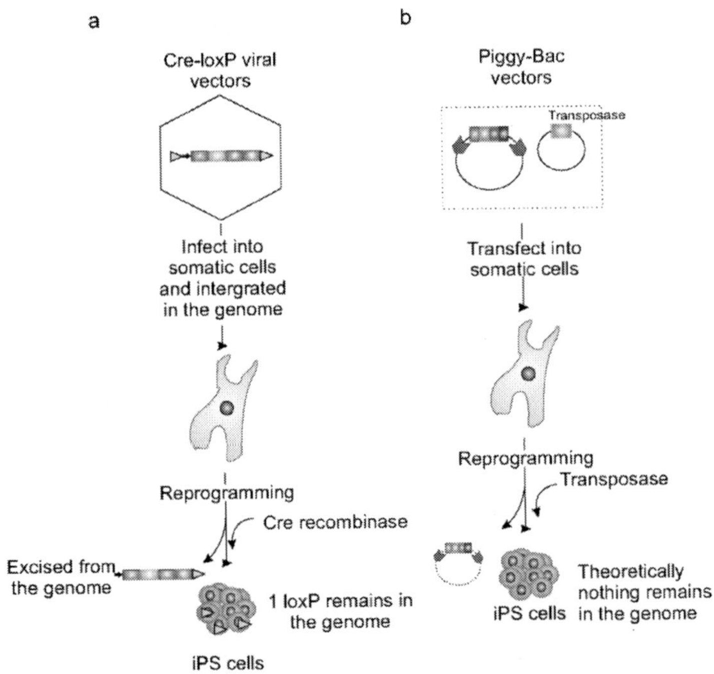

Figure 3. Methods for production of induced pluripotent stem cells (iPSCs) by excisable integrating vectors. Two different methods exist today to generate iPSCs by excisable integrating vectors: by Cre-loxP and Piggy-Bac vectors. a) In the Cre-loxP viral delivery system, defined reprogramming factors are cloned into vectors flanked by recognition sites, loxP sites, for Crerecombinase. Upon transduction into somatic cells, the loxP site is duplicated and reprogramming factos are stably integrated into the genome flanked by loxP sites. When Crerecombinase is expressed, the integrated reprogramming factors are excised from the genome but one loxP site is left behind integrated into the genome of iPSCs. b) The Piggy-Bac transposon gene delivery system is based on a mobile genetic element that efficiently integrates into the genome of mammalian cells. When fusion gene encoding defined reprogramming factors in the transposon expression vector as well as transposase expression vector are transfected into somatic cells, the fusion gene is stably integrated into the genome. When transposase is expressed, the interated genetic material is excised from the genome resulting in transgene- and vector free iPSCs.

Taken together, all these improvements mark important steps towards the generation of more efficient and safer iPSCs.

Other Methods to Achieve Reprogramming - 1.Cloning = Somatic Cell Nuclear Transfer (SCNT) 2.Cell Fusion 3.Egg Extract

In addition to the iPS procedure other ways exist to reprogram somatic cells including: 1) somatic cell nuclear transfer (SCNT), 2) cell fusion of somatic adult cells with pluripotent ESCs to generate hybrid cells and 3) cell extract from ESCs or embryo carcinoma cells (ECs). From the time when successful SCNT experiments, more commonly known as cloning, in the frog *Xenopus Laevis* (Gurdon et al., 1958) to the creation of the sheep Dolly (Wilmut et al., 1997), it has been proven that an adult cell nucleus transplanted into an unfertilized egg can support development into a new individual, and researchers have focused on identifying the molecular mechanisms that take place during this remarkable process. Even though SCNT has been around for 50 years, the molecular mechanisms that take place inside the egg remain unknown. This is largely attributed to the fact that only one tiny nucleus is placed inside an in comparison to gigantic egg cell, which is in itself difficult to knock out genes in. It requires single cell analysis approaches in the huge background noise that the egg cytoplasm represent. In 2007 a report that the first primate ESCs were isolated from SCNT blastula embryos of the species Rhesus Monkey was published (Byrne et al., 2007). The reason why it took so long to perform successful SCNT in Rhesus Monkey was a technical issue; to enucleate the egg, modified polarized light was used instead of traditional methods using either mechanical removal of DNA or UV light mediated DNA destruction. The first reliable publication of successful human SCNT reported generation of a single cloned blastocyst (Stojkovic et al., 2005). Unfortunately, dramatic advances in human SCNT reported by Hwang and colleagues in South Korea were largely a product of fraud (Cho et al., 2006). In human SCNT reports, left over eggs from IVF (*in vitro* fertilization) that failed to fertilize have been used, indicating poor egg quality. Remarkably, human SCNT using 29 donated eggs (oocytes) of good quality, and not leftovers from IVF, from three young women were reported to develop into cloned blastocysts, at a frequency as high as 23% (French et al., 2008). Theoretically, human embryonic stem cells (hESCs) can be derived *in vitro* from SCNT generated blastocysts. These patient-specific hESCs can multiply in tissue culture and upon external signals be differentiated into any cell type in the body, which could be transplanted to patients suffering from disease. Those cells could also be used as a human *in vitro* model system to test patient specific developmental pathways and pharmaceutical products. However, so far no established hESC line using the SCNT procedure has been reported. The shortage of donated high quality human eggs for research is a significant impediment for this field.

Fusion of somatic adult cells with pluripotent ESCs to generate hybrid cells or using cell extract from ESCs or ECs have been used to reprogram different cell types into a transient ESC-like state (Bhutani et al., 2010; Cowan et al., 2005; Freberg et al., 2007; Taranger et al., 2005; Yamanaka and Blau, 2010) and are other methods that have been used to elucidate the molecular mechanism of reprogramming.

Mechanisms of Reprogramming

The crucial event during reprogramming is the activation of ES- and the silencing of differentiation- markers, while the genetic code remains intact. Major reprogramming of gene expression takes place inside the egg and genes that have been silenced during embryo development are awakened. In contrast, genes that are expressed in, and are specific for, the donated cell nucleus become inactivated most of the times, however some SCNT embryos remember their heritage and fail to inactivate somatic-specific genes (Ng and Gurdon, 2008). It has been reported that reprogramming involves changes in chromatin structure and chromatin components (Jullien et al., 2010; Kikyo et al., 2000). Importantly, initiation of Oct4 expression has been found to be crucial for successful nuclear transfers (Boiani et al., 2002; Byrne et al., 2003) and important for iPSC creation; all other reprogramming iPSC transcription factors have been replaced with other factors or chemical compounds, but only one report so far could exclude Oct4. In murine ES cells, Oct4 must hold a precise level to maintain them as just ES cells (Niwa et al., 2000) and therefore understanding the control of the Oct4 level will be key if one wants to understand pluripotency and reprogramming at the molecular level. Recent report demonstrated that Oct4 expression is regulated by SAF-A. SAF-A was found on the Oct4 promoter only when the gene is actively transcribed in murine ESCs, depending on LIF and gene silencing of SAF-A in ESCs resulted in down regulation of Oct4 (Vizlin-Hodzic et al., 2011). Other Oct4 modulators have been reported that in similarity with SAF-A are in complex with RNA polymerase II (Ding et al., 2009; Ponnusamy et al., 2009). Post-translational modifications have been shown to be able to modify the activity of Oct4, such as sumoylation (Wei et al., 2007) and ubiquitination (Xu et al., 2004). During the reprogramming process epigenetic marks are changed. Removal of methyl groups on DNA (DNA demethylation) of the Oct4 promoter has been shown to occur in frog oocytes (Simonsson and Gurdon, 2004) and demethylation has been observed in mouse (Yamazaki et al., 2006) during SCNT. The growth arrest and DNA damage inducible protein Gadd45a was shown to promote DNA demethylation (Barreto et al., 2007), suggesting that DNA demethylation is occurring by a DNA repair mechanism. Recently in cell fusion experiments the deaminase Aid was identified to play a role in demethylation of the Oct4 and Nanog promoters (Bhutani et al., 2010). Consistent with those findings is that Aid together with Gadd45 and Mbd4 has been shown to promote DNA demethylation in zebrafish (Rai et al., 2008). Translational tumor protein (Tpt1) has been proposed to control Oct4 and shown to interact with nucleophosmin (Npm1) during mitosis of ESCs and such complexes are involved in cell proliferation (Johansson et al., 2010b; Koziol et al., 2007). Furthermore, phosphorylated nucleolin (Ncl-P) interacts with Oct4 during interphase in both murine and human ESCs (Johansson et al., 2010a). Core transcription factors, Oct4, Sox2 and Nanog, were shown to individually form complexes with nucleophosmin (Npm1) to control ESCs (Johansson and Simonsson, 2010). ESCs also display high levels of telomerase activity which maintain the length of the telomeres. The telomerase activity or Tert gene expression is rapidly down regulated during differentiation and are much lower or absent in somatic cells. Therefore, reestablishment of high telomerase activity (or reactivation of Tert gene) is important for reprogramming. In SCNT animals, telomere length in somatic cells has been reported to be comparable to that in normally fertilized animals (Betts et al., 2001; Lanza et al., 2000; Tian et al., 2000). Recently, a telomere length-resetting mechanism has been identified in the *Xenopus* egg (Vizlin-Hodzic et al., 2009).

When iPSCs first were introduced many thought that the molecular mechanism of reprogramming was solved once and for all. It was soon shown that to generate iPSC colonies one could use different combinations of transcription factors most efficiently together with retroviruses or more recently, exposure to chemical compounds together with the transcription factors, Oct4 and KLf4, and with retroviruses (Zhu et al., 2010) or retroviruses alone (Kane et al., 2010). What retroviruses do for the reprogramming process is unknown and the efficiency by which egg reprograms the somatic cells is far more efficient than the iPSC procedure. Moreover, mutagenic effects have been documented in both laboratory and clinical gene therapy studies, principally as a result of a dysregulated host gene expression in the proximity of gene integration sites. So the first question to ask is whether all iPSC experiments so far forgot the obvious control of using only virus. The answer is probably no because the efficiency is very low with viruses alone as compared to using transcription factors combined with virus or identified reprogramming compounds. Reprogramming an adult somatic frog cell nucleus to generate a normal "clonal" new individual is far less efficient (0.1-3%) than reprogramming to create a blastocyst, from which ESCs are isolated (efficiency 20-40%) (Gurdon, 2008) and is comparable with blastula formation after human SCNT (23%). This number could be compared with iPSC procedure that has reported 0.5 % success rate at most with human cells (table 1). The low efficiency and slow kinetics of iPSC derivation suggest that there are other procedures that are more efficient, yet to decipher. There is a belief that there are different levels of pluripotency when it comes to ESC and also that reprogramming follows an organized sequence of events, beginning with downregulation of somatic markers and activation of pluripotency markers SSEA-1, alkaline phosphatase, and Fbxo15 before pluripotency endogenous genes such as Oct4 and Nanog become expressed and cells gain independence from exogenous transcription factor expression (Brambrink et al., 2008; Stadtfeld et al., 2008a). Only a small subset of somatic cells expressing the reprogramming factors down-regulates somatic markers and activates pluripotency genes (Wernig et al., 2008a).

History of Reprogramming

SCNT has been around for more than fifty years although it was already proposed in 1938 by Hans Spemann (Spemann, 1938), an embryologist who received the Nobel Prize in Medicine for his development of new embryological micro surgery techniques. Spemann anticipated that "transplanting an older nucleus into an egg would be a fantastic experiment". Later on, Robert Briggs and Thomas King were the first to put the nuclear transfer technique into practice. However, they only managed to obtain viable offspring through nuclear transfer of undifferentiated cells in the frog species *Rana pipiens* (Briggs and King, 1952). During the 1950s to the 1970s a series of pioneering somatic nuclear transfer experiments performed by John Gurdon showed that nuclei from differentiated amphibian cells, such as tadpole intestinal or adult skin cells could generate cloned tadpoles (Gurdon, 1962; Gurdon et al., 1958; Gurdon et al., 1975). In 1997, the successful cloning of a mammal was first achieved. The sheep Dolly was produced by using the nuclei of cells cultured from an adult mammary gland (Wilmut et al., 1997). Following the cloning of Dolly, researchers have reported successful cloning of a number of species including cow, pig, mouse, rabbit, cat (named Copycat) and monkey. In 2006, reprogrammed murine iPSCs were reported by Takahashi and Yamanaka (Takahashi and Yamanaka, 2006) and in 2007 human iPSCs were reported (Takahashi et al., 2007; Yu et al., 2009).

Transplanting Cells

In order to make cell therapy (route 1 in Figure 1) using iPSCs a reality in medicine many obstacles need to be overcome. Organ transplantation between individuals is complicated due to the limited availability of matched tissues and consequently the requirement for life-long treatment with immunosuppressive drugs that can cause serious side effects. The hope is that iPSCs that are already genetically matched with the patient would circumvent these issues. Another advantage of iPSCs over current transplantation approaches is the opportunity of repairing mutations that cause the disease by homologous recombination, which has not been very successful in adult stem cells due to difficulties in propagating those cells *in vitro*. In mouse, iPSC technology combined with correction of a known disease-causing mutation has been proven successful. In human autologous cell therapy has been used since the mid 90′s for the treatment of focal cartilage lesions, using the patient's chondrocytes transplanted into the injured knee (Brittberg et al., 1994), thereby alleviated osteoarthritic symptoms and induction of tissue repair. The cell therapy gives stable long-term results up to 20 years after surgery in some patients but is less successful in others (Lindahl et al., 2003; Peterson et al., 2010). One drawback with this technique is the supply of cells. Large injuries require large amounts of cells, and there is a limit of the size the biopsies that can be taken out from the patient. Introducing the iPSC technique in such system might improve the process. Since the iPSC have theoretically an unlimited proliferation capacity, these cells can be used to reach larger quantities of cells. When sufficient numbers have been produced, the iPSC are differentiated into chondrocytes and transplanted to the lesion. In this case, no biopsy would need to be harvested, since iPSC can be made from a regular skin fibroblast. Before this somewhat futuristic scenario can come true, rigorous characterization of the iPSC is needed, since these cells, as all stem cells, can form terratoma *in vivo* (Fairchild, 2010). The iPSC have however, been shown to retain their epigenic memory from the tissue which they originate. It would therefore be easier to differentiate an iPSC to a chondrocyte if the donor cell was a chondrocyte (Kim et al., 2010), and maybe terminally so, thus avoiding risk for terratoma formation. A biopsy would thus be needed, but a relatively small cell harvest could with the iPSC technique result in the treatment of larger injuries. The iPSC procedure could also lead to a therapy-outcome that is more predicted and constant due to that chondrogenic differentiation of iPSC probably result in a more homogeneous cell-lineage.

Direct Programming of Somatic Cells Into Another Cell Type

Switching from one somatic cell type into another cell type, not necessarily via a pluripotent cell state was first demonstrated when fibroblasts formed myofibers after transduction with retroviral vectors expressing the skeletal muscle factor MyoD (Davis et al., 1987). Further, it has been reported that pancreatic acinar cells could be transformed into insulin-producing β cells by overexpression of the pancreatic factors Pdx1, MafA and Ngn3 *in vivo* (Zhou et al., 2008) as well as that ESCs could be directly differentiated into specific dopamine neurons by overexpression of only one factor, Lmx1 (Friling et al., 2009). These experiments proved that transdifferentiation do not require reprogramming into a pluripotent state, although all such experiments have used some kind of retroviruses and if only virus in itself can contribute to pluripotency as has recently been shown one cannot completely rule out that the switch hasn't passed via a pluripotent state.

Final Remarks

Some will argue that the complexity of reprogramming is solved by the iPSC technology, however apart from the defined reprogramming factors, retroviruses help in the reprogramming process in an unknown way, and is still inefficient compared to SCNT which argues for that more can be learnt about reprogramming. Also the fact that different combinations of reprogramming factors, or replacement with chemicals, have been used successfully indicates that there exist reprogramming molecules yet to be discovered. Therefore, further investigations are needed to learn more about the molecular mechanisms of iPSCs and how to prevent tumor formation following *in vivo* transplantation. Awaiting *in vivo* safety, these techniques offer exciting possibilities for mapping mechanisms of different diseases and screening for patient-specific therapies and drugs. To derive iPSCs from the patient's own cells following differentiation into the disease-causing cells means recapitulating the disease in a test tube for genomic, proteomic and epigenomic analysis. The iPSC as a human *in vitro* disease modeling system is a new promising and fast expanding research area.

References

Aasen, T., Raya, A., Barrero, M.J., Garreta, E., Consiglio, A., Gonzalez, F., Vassena, R., Bilic, J., Pekarik, V., Tiscornia, G., *et al.* (2008). Efficient and rapid generation of induced pluripotent stem cells from human keratinocytes. *Nat Biotechnol 26*, 1276-1284.

Aoki, T., Ohnishi, H., Oda, Y., Tadokoro, M., Sasao, M., Kato, H., Hattori, K., and Ohgushi, H. (2010). Generation of induced pluripotent stem cells from human adipose-derived stem cells without c-MYC. *Tissue Eng Part A 16*, 2197-2206.

Barreto, G., Schafer, A., Marhold, J., Stach, D., Swaminathan, S.K., Handa, V., Doderlein, G., Maltry, N., Wu, W., Lyko, F., *et al.* (2007). Gadd45a promotes epigenetic gene activation by repair-mediated DNA demethylation. *Nature 445*, 671-675.

Bass, A.J., Watanabe, H., Mermel, C.H., Yu, S., Perner, S., Verhaak, R.G., Kim, S.Y., Wardwell, L., Tamayo, P., Gat-Viks, I., *et al.* (2009). SOX2 is an amplified lineage-survival oncogene in lung and esophageal squamous cell carcinomas. *Nat Genet 41*, 1238-1242.

Betts, D., Bordignon, V., Hill, J., Winger, Q., Westhusin, M., Smith, L., and King, W. (2001). Reprogramming of telomerase activity and rebuilding of telomere length in cloned cattle. *Proc Natl Acad Sci U S A 98*, 1077-1082.

Bhutani, N., Brady, J.J., Damian, M., Sacco, A., Corbel, S.Y., and Blau, H.M. (2010). Reprogramming towards pluripotency requires AID-dependent DNA demethylation. *Nature 463*, 1042-1047.

Boiani, M., Eckardt, S., Scholer, H.R., and McLaughlin, K.J. (2002). Oct4 distribution and level in mouse clones: consequences for pluripotency. *Genes Dev 16*, 1209-1219.

Brambrink, T., Foreman, R., Welstead, G.G., Lengner, C.J., Wernig, M., Suh, H., and Jaenisch, R. (2008). Sequential expression of pluripotency markers during direct reprogramming of mouse somatic cells. *Cell Stem Cell 2*, 151-159.

Briggs, R., and King, T.J. (1952). Transplantation of Living Nuclei From Blastula Cells into Enucleated Frogs' Eggs. *Proc Natl Acad Sci U S A 38*, 455-463.

Brittberg, M., Lindahl, A., Nilsson, A., Ohlsson, C., Isaksson, O., and Peterson, L. (1994). Treatment of deep cartilage defects in the knee with autologous chondrocyte transplantation. *N Engl J Med 331*, 889-895.

Byrne, J.A., Pedersen, D.A., Clepper, L.L., Nelson, M., Sanger, W.G., Gokhale, S., Wolf, D.P., and Mitalipov, S.M. (2007). Producing primate embryonic stem cells by somatic cell nuclear transfer. *Nature 450*, 497-502.

Byrne, J.A., Simonsson, S., Western, P.S., and Gurdon, J.B. (2003). Nuclei of adult mammalian somatic cells are directly reprogrammed to oct-4 stem cell gene expression by amphibian oocytes. *Curr Biol 13*, 1206-1213.

Chang, C.W., Lai, Y.S., Pawlik, K.M., Liu, K., Sun, C.W., Li, C., Schoeb, T.R., and Townes, T.M. (2009). Polycistronic lentiviral vector for "hit and run" reprogramming of adult skin fibroblasts to induced pluripotent stem cells. *Stem Cells 27*, 1042-1049.

Cho, M.K., McGee, G., and Magnus, D. (2006). Research conduct. Lessons of the stem cell scandal. *Science 311*, 614-615.

Cowan, C.A., Atienza, J., Melton, D.A., and Eggan, K. (2005). Nuclear reprogramming of somatic cells after fusion with human embryonic stem cells. *Science 309*, 1369-1373.

Davis, R.L., Weintraub, H., and Lassar, A.B. (1987). Expression of a single transfected cDNA converts fibroblasts to myoblasts. *Cell 51*, 987-1000.

Dimos, J.T., Rodolfa, K.T., Niakan, K.K., Weisenthal, L.M., Mitsumoto, H., Chung, W., Croft, G.F., Saphier, G., Leibel, R., Goland, R., *et al.* (2008).

Induced pluripotent stem cells generated from patients with ALS can be differentiated into motor neurons. *Science 321*, 1218-1221.

Ding, L., Paszkowski-Rogacz, M., Nitzsche, A., Slabicki, M.M., Heninger, A.K., de Vries, I., Kittler, R., Junqueira, M., Shevchenko, A., Schulz, H., *et al.* (2009). A genome-scale RNAi screen for Oct4 modulators defines a role of the Paf1 complex for embryonic stem cell identity. *Cell Stem Cell 4*, 403-415.

Eminli, S., Foudi, A., Stadtfeld, M., Maherali, N., Ahfeldt, T., Mostoslavsky, G., Hock, H., and Hochedlinger, K. (2009). Differentiation stage determines potential of hematopoietic cells for reprogramming into induced pluripotent stem cells. *Nat Genet 41*, 968-976.

Fairchild, P.J. (2010). The challenge of immunogenicity in the quest for induced pluripotency. *Nat Rev Immunol 10*, 868-875.

Freberg, C.T., Dahl, J.A., Timoskainen, S., and Collas, P. (2007). Epigenetic reprogramming of OCT4 and NANOG regulatory regions by embryonal carcinoma cell extract. *Mol Biol Cell 18*, 1543-1553.

French, A.J., Adams, C.A., Anderson, L.S., Kitchen, J.R., Hughes, M.R., and Wood, S.H. (2008). Development of human cloned blastocysts following somatic cell nuclear transfer with adult fibroblasts. *Stem Cells 26*, 485-493.

Friling, S., Andersson, E., Thompson, L.H., Jonsson, M.E., Hebsgaard, J.B., Nanou, E., Alekseenko, Z., Marklund, U., Kjellander, S., Volakakis, N., *et al.* (2009). Efficient production of mesencephalic dopamine neurons by Lmx1a expression in embryonic stem cells. *Proc Natl Acad Sci U S A 106*, 7613-7618.

Gidekel, S., Pizov, G., Bergman, Y., and Pikarsky, E. (2003). Oct-3/4 is a dose-dependent oncogenic fate determinant. *Cancer Cell 4*, 361-370.

Giorgetti, A., Montserrat, N., Aasen, T., Gonzalez, F., Rodriguez-Piza, I., Vassena, R., Raya, A., Boue, S., Barrero, M.J., Corbella, B.A., *et al.* (2009). Generation of induced pluripotent stem cells from human cord blood using OCT4 and SOX2. *Cell Stem Cell 5*, 353-357.

Gonzalez, F., Barragan Monasterio, M., Tiscornia, G., Montserrat Pulido, N., Vassena, R., Batlle Morera, L., Rodriguez Piza, I., and Izpisua Belmonte, J.C. (2009). Generation of mouse-induced pluripotent stem cells by transient expression of a single nonviral polycistronic vector. *Proc Natl Acad Sci U S A 106*, 8918-8922.

Gurdon, J. (2008). Primate therapeutic cloning in practice. *Nat Biotechnol 26*, 64-65.

Gurdon, J.B. (1962). The developmental capacity of nuclei taken from intestinal epithelium cells of feeding tadpoles. *J Embryol Exp Morphol 10*, 622-640.

Gurdon, J.B., Elsdale, T.R., and Fischberg, M. (1958). Sexually mature individuals of Xenopus laevis from the transplantation of single somatic nuclei. *Nature 182*, 64-65.

Gurdon, J.B., Laskey, R.A., and Reeves, O.R. (1975). The developmental capacity of nuclei transplanted from keratinized skin cells of adult frogs. *J Embryol Exp Morphol 34*, 93-112.

Haase, A., Olmer, R., Schwanke, K., Wunderlich, S., Merkert, S., Hess, C., Zweigerdt, R., Gruh, I., Meyer, J., Wagner, S., *et al.* (2009). Generation of induced pluripotent stem cells from human cord blood. *Cell Stem Cell 5*, 434-441.

Hanna, J., Wernig, M., Markoulaki, S., Sun, C.W., Meissner, A., Cassady, J.P., Beard, C., Brambrink, T., Wu, L.C., Townes, T.M., *et al.* (2007). Treatment of sickle cell anemia mouse model with iPS cells generated from autologous skin. *Science 318*, 1920-1923.

Heng, J.C., Feng, B., Han, J., Jiang, J., Kraus, P., Ng, J.H., Orlov, Y.L., Huss, M., Yang, L., Lufkin, T., *et al.* (2010). The nuclear receptor Nr5a2 can replace Oct4 in the reprogramming of murine somatic cells to pluripotent cells. *Cell Stem Cell 6*, 167-174.

Huangfu, D., Maehr, R., Guo, W., Eijkelenboom, A., Snitow, M., Chen, A.E., and Melton, D.A. (2008a). Induction of pluripotent stem cells by defined factors is greatly improved by small-molecule compounds. *Nat Biotechnol 26*, 795-797.

Huangfu, D., Osafune, K., Maehr, R., Guo, W., Eijkelenboom, A., Chen, S., Muhlestein, W., and Melton, D.A. (2008b). Induction of pluripotent stem cells from primary human fibroblasts with only Oct4 and Sox2. *Nat Biotechnol 26*, 1269-1275.

Jia, F., Wilson, K.D., Sun, N., Gupta, D.M., Huang, M., Li, Z., Panetta, N.J., Chen, Z.Y., Robbins, R.C., Kay, M.A., *et al.* (2010). A nonviral minicircle vector for deriving human iPS cells. *Nat Methods 7*, 197-199.

Johansson, H., and Simonsson, S. (2010). Core transcription factors, Oct4, Sox2 and Nanog, individually form complexes with nucleophosmin (Npm1) to control embryonic stem (ES) cell fate determination. *Aging (*Albany NY) *2*, 815-822.

Johansson, H., Svensson, F., Runnberg, R., Simonsson, T., and Simonsson, S. (2010a). Phosphorylated nucleolin interacts with translationally controlled tumor protein during mitosis and with Oct4 during interphase in ES cells. *PLoS One 5*, e13678.

Johansson, H., Vizlin-Hodzic, D., Simonsson, T., and Simonsson, S. (2010b). Translationally controlled tumor protein interacts with nucleophosmin during mitosis in ES cells. *Cell Cycle 9.*

Jullien, J., Astrand, C., Halley-Stott, R.P., Garrett, N., and Gurdon, J.B. (2010). Characterization of somatic cell nuclear reprogramming by oocytes in which a linker histone is required for pluripotency gene reactivation. *Proc Natl Acad Sci U S A 107*, 5483-5488.

Kane, N.M., Nowrouzi, A., Mukherjee, S., Blundell, M.P., Greig, J.A., Lee, W.K., Houslay, M.D., Milligan, G., Mountford, J.C., von Kalle, C., *et al.* (2010). Lentivirus-mediated reprogramming of somatic cells in the absence of transgenic transcription factors. *Mol Ther 18*, 2139-2145.

Kazuki, Y., Hiratsuka, M., Takiguchi, M., Osaki, M., Kajitani, N., Hoshiya, H., Hiramatsu, K., Yoshino, T., Kazuki, K., Ishihara, C., *et al.* (2010). Complete genetic correction of ips cells from Duchenne muscular dystrophy. *Mol Ther 18*, 386-393.

Kikyo, N., Wade, P.A., Guschin, D., Ge, H., and Wolffe, A.P. (2000). Active remodeling of somatic nuclei in egg cytoplasm by the nucleosomal ATPase ISWI. *Science 289*, 2360-2362.

Kim, J.B., Zaehres, H., Wu, G., Gentile, L., Ko, K., Sebastiano, V., Arauzo-Bravo, M.J., Ruau, D., Han, D.W., Zenke, M., *et al.* (2008). Pluripotent stem cells induced from adult neural stem cells by reprogramming with two factors. *Nature 454*, 646-650.

Kim, K., Doi, A., Wen, B., Ng, K., Zhao, R., Cahan, P., Kim, J., Aryee, M.J., Ji, H., Ehrlich, L.I., *et al.* (2010). Epigenetic memory in induced pluripotent stem cells. *Nature 467*, 285-290.

Koziol, M.J., Garrett, N., and Gurdon, J.B. (2007). Tpt1 activates transcription of oct4 and nanog in transplanted somatic nuclei. *Curr Biol 17*, 801-807.

Lanza, R.P., Cibelli, J.B., Blackwell, C., Cristofalo, V.J., Francis, M.K., Baerlocher, G.M., Mak, J., Schertzer, M., Chavez, E.A., Sawyer, N., *et al.* (2000). Extension of cell life-span and telomere length in animals cloned from senescent somatic cells. *Science 288*, 665-669.

Li, C., Zhou, J., Shi, G., Ma, Y., Yang, Y., Gu, J., Yu, H., Jin, S., Wei, Z., Chen, F., *et al.* (2009). Pluripotency can be rapidly and efficiently induced in human amniotic fluid-derived cells. *Hum Mol Genet 18*, 4340-4349.

Lindahl, A., Brittberg, M., and Peterson, L. (2003). Cartilage repair with chondrocytes: clinical and cellular aspects. *Novartis Found Symp 249*, 175-186; discussion 186-179, 234-178, 239-141.

Liu, H., Ye, Z., Kim, Y., Sharkis, S., and Jang, Y.Y. (2010). Generation of endoderm-derived human induced pluripotent stem cells from primary hepatocytes. *Hepatology 51*, 1810-1819.

Loh, Y.H., Agarwal, S., Park, I.H., Urbach, A., Huo, H., Heffner, G.C., Kim, K., Miller, J.D., Ng, K., and Daley, G.Q. (2009). Generation of induced pluripotent stem cells from human blood. *Blood 113*, 5476-5479.

Lowry, W.E., Richter, L., Yachechko, R., Pyle, A.D., Tchieu, J., Sridharan, R., Clark, A.T., and Plath, K. (2008). Generation of human induced pluripotent stem cells from dermal fibroblasts. *Proc Natl Acad Sci U S A 105*, 2883-2888.

Meissner, A., Wernig, M., and Jaenisch, R. (2007). Direct reprogramming of genetically unmodified fibroblasts into pluripotent stem cells. *Nat Biotechnol 25*, 1177-1181.

Nakagawa, M., Koyanagi, M., Tanabe, K., Takahashi, K., Ichisaka, T., Aoi, T., Okita, K., Mochiduki, Y., Takizawa, N., and Yamanaka, S. (2008). Generation of induced pluripotent stem cells without Myc from mouse and human fibroblasts. *Nat Biotechnol 26*, 101-106.

Ng, R.K., and Gurdon, J.B. (2008). Epigenetic memory of an active gene state depends on histone H3.3 incorporation into chromatin in the absence of transcription. *Nat Cell Biol 10*, 102-109.

Niwa, H., Miyazaki, J., and Smith, A.G. (2000). Quantitative expression of Oct-3/4 defines differentiation, dedifferentiation or self-renewal of ES cells. *Nat Genet 24*, 372-376.

Okita, K., Ichisaka, T., and Yamanaka, S. (2007). Generation of germline-competent induced pluripotent stem cells. *Nature 448*, 313-317.

Okita, K., Nakagawa, M., Hyenjong, H., Ichisaka, T., and Yamanaka, S. (2008). Generation of mouse induced pluripotent stem cells without viral vectors. *Science 322*, 949-953.

Park, I.H., Arora, N., Huo, H., Maherali, N., Ahfeldt, T., Shimamura, A., Lensch, M.W., Cowan, C., Hochedlinger, K., and Daley, G.Q. (2008a). Disease-specific induced pluripotent stem cells. *Cell 134*, 877-886.

Park, I.H., Zhao, R., West, J.A., Yabuuchi, A., Huo, H., Ince, T.A., Lerou, P.H., Lensch, M.W., and Daley, G.Q. (2008b). Reprogramming of human somatic cells to pluripotency with defined factors. *Nature 451*, 141-146.

Peterson, L., Vasiliadis, H.S., Brittberg, M., and Lindahl, A. (2010). Autologous chondrocyte implantation: a long-term follow-up. *Am J Sports Med 38*, 1117-1124.

Ponnusamy, M.P., Deb, S., Dey, P., Chakraborty, S., Rachagani, S., Senapati, S., and Batra, S.K. (2009). RNA polymerase II associated factor 1/PD2 maintains self-renewal by its interaction with Oct3/4 in mouse embryonic stem cells. *Stem Cells 27*, 3001-3011.

Rai, K., Huggins, I.J., James, S.R., Karpf, A.R., Jones, D.A., and Cairns, B.R. (2008). DNA demethylation in zebrafish involves the coupling of a deaminase, a glycosylase, and gadd45. *Cell 135*, 1201-1212.

Shi, Y., Do, J.T., Desponts, C., Hahm, H.S., Scholer, H.R., and Ding, S. (2008). A combined chemical and genetic approach for the generation of induced pluripotent stem cells. *Cell Stem Cell 2*, 525-528.

Silva, J., Barrandon, O., Nichols, J., Kawaguchi, J., Theunissen, T.W., and Smith, A. (2008). Promotion of reprogramming to ground state pluripotency by signal inhibition. *PLoS Biol 6, e253.*

Simonsson, S., and Gurdon, J. (2004). DNA demethylation is necessary for the epigenetic reprogramming of somatic cell nuclei. *Nat Cell Biol 6*, 984-990.

Soldner, F., Hockemeyer, D., Beard, C., Gao, Q., Bell, G.W., Cook, E.G., Hargus, G., Blak, A., Cooper, O., Mitalipova, M., *et al.* (2009). Parkinson's disease patient-derived induced pluripotent stem cells free of viral reprogramming factors. *Cell 136*, 964-977.

Spemann, H. (1938). *Embryonic Development and Induction*. New Haven: Yale University Press.

Stadtfeld, M., Maherali, N., Breault, D.T., and Hochedlinger, K. (2008a). Defining molecular cornerstones during fibroblast to iPS cell reprogramming in mouse. *Cell Stem Cell 2*, 230-240.

Stadtfeld, M., Nagaya, M., Utikal, J., Weir, G., and Hochedlinger, K. (2008b). Induced pluripotent stem cells generated without viral integration. *Science 322*, 945-949.

Stojkovic, M., Stojkovic, P., Leary, C., Hall, V.J., Armstrong, L., Herbert, M., Nesbitt, M., Lako, M., and Murdoch, A. (2005). Derivation of a human blastocyst after heterologous nuclear transfer to donated oocytes. *Reprod Biomed Online 11*, 226-231.

Sugii, S., Kida, Y., Kawamura, T., Suzuki, J., Vassena, R., Yin, Y.Q., Lutz, M.K., Berggren, W.T., Izpisua Belmonte, J.C., and Evans, R.M. (2010). Human and mouse adipose-derived cells support feeder-independent induction of pluripotent stem cells. *Proc Natl Acad Sci U S A 107*, 3558-3563.

Takahashi, K., Tanabe, K., Ohnuki, M., Narita, M., Ichisaka, T., Tomoda, K., and Yamanaka, S. (2007). Induction of pluripotent stem cells from adult human fibroblasts by defined factors. *Cell 131*, 861-872.

Takahashi, K., and Yamanaka, S. (2006). Induction of pluripotent stem cells from mouse embryonic and adult fibroblast cultures by defined factors. *Cell 126*, 663-676.

Taranger, C.K., Noer, A., Sorensen, A.L., Hakelien, A.M., Boquest, A.C., and Collas, P. (2005). Induction of dedifferentiation, genomewide transcriptional programming, and epigenetic reprogramming by extracts of carcinoma and embryonic stem cells. *Mol Biol Cell 16*, 5719-5735.

Tian, X.C., Xu, J., and Yang, X. (2000). Normal telomere lengths found in cloned cattle. *Nat Genet 26*, 272-273.

Tsai, S.Y., Clavel, C., Kim, S., Ang, Y.S., Grisanti, L., Lee, D.F., Kelley, K., and Rendl, M. (2010). Oct4 and klf4 reprogram dermal papilla cells into induced pluripotent stem cells. *Stem Cells 28*, 221-228.

Vizlin-Hodzic, D., Johansson, H., Ryme, J., Simonsson, T., and Simonsson, S. (2011). SAF-A Has a Role in Transcriptional Regulation of Oct4 in ES Cells Through Promoter Binding. *Cell Reprogram.*

Vizlin-Hodzic, D., Ryme, J., Simonsson, S., and Simonsson, T. (2009). Developmental studies of Xenopus shelterin complexes: the message to reset telomere length is already present in the egg. *FASEB J 23*, 2587-2594.

Wei, D., Kanai, M., Huang, S., and Xie, K. (2006). Emerging role of KLF4 in human gastrointestinal cancer. *Carcinogenesis 27*, 23-31.

Wei, F., Scholer, H.R., and Atchison, M.L. (2007). Sumoylation of Oct4 enhances its stability, DNA binding, and transactivation. *J Biol Chem 282*, 21551-21560.

Wernig, M., Lengner, C.J., Hanna, J., Lodato, M.A., Steine, E., Foreman, R., Staerk, J., Markoulaki, S., and Jaenisch, R. (2008a). A drug-inducible transgenic system for direct reprogramming of multiple somatic cell types. *Nat Biotechnol 26*, 916-924.

Wernig, M., Meissner, A., Cassady, J.P., and Jaenisch, R. (2008b). c-Myc is dispensable for direct reprogramming of mouse fibroblasts. *Cell Stem Cell 2*, 10-12.

Wernig, M., Meissner, A., Foreman, R., Brambrink, T., Ku, M., Hochedlinger, K., Bernstein, B.E., and Jaenisch, R. (2007). In vitro reprogramming of fibroblasts into a pluripotent ES-cell-like state. *Nature 448*, 318-324.

Wernig, M., Zhao, J.P., Pruszak, J., Hedlund, E., Fu, D., Soldner, F., Broccoli, V., Constantine-Paton, M., Isacson, O., and Jaenisch, R. (2008c). Neurons derived from reprogrammed fibroblasts functionally integrate into the fetal brain and improve symptoms of rats with Parkinson's disease. *Proc Natl Acad Sci U S A 105*, 5856-5861.

Wilmut, I., Schnieke, A.E., McWhir, J., Kind, A.J., and Campbell, K.H. (1997). Viable offspring derived from fetal and adult mammalian cells. *Nature 385*, 810-813.

Woltjen, K., Michael, I.P., Mohseni, P., Desai, R., Mileikovsky, M., Hamalainen, R., Cowling, R., Wang, W., Liu, P., Gertsenstein, M., *et al.* (2009). piggyBac transposition reprograms fibroblasts to induced pluripotent stem cells. *Nature 458*, 766-770.

Xu, D., Alipio, Z., Fink, L.M., Adcock, D.M., Yang, J., Ward, D.C., and Ma, Y. (2009). Phenotypic correction of murine hemophilia A using an iPS cell-based therapy. *Proc Natl Acad Sci U S A 106*, 808-813.

Xu, H.M., Liao, B., Zhang, Q.J., Wang, B.B., Li, H., Zhong, X.M., Sheng, H.Z., Zhao, Y.X., Zhao, Y.M., and Jin, Y. (2004). Wwp2, an E3 ubiquitin ligase that targets transcription factor Oct-4 for ubiquitination. *J Biol Chem 279*, 23495-23503.

Yamanaka, S. (2009). A fresh look at iPS cells. *Cell 137*, 13-17.

Yamanaka, S., and Blau, H.M. (2010). Nuclear reprogramming to a pluripotent state by three approaches. *Nature 465*, 704-712.

Yamazaki, Y., Fujita, T.C., Low, E.W., Alarcon, V.B., Yanagimachi, R., and Marikawa, Y. (2006). Gradual DNA demethylation of the Oct4 promoter in cloned mouse embryos. *Mol Reprod Dev 73*, 180-188.

Yu, J., Hu, K., Smuga-Otto, K., Tian, S., Stewart, R., Slukvin, II, and Thomson, J.A. (2009). Human induced pluripotent stem cells free of vector and transgene sequences. *Science 324*, 797-801.

Yu, J., Vodyanik, M.A., Smuga-Otto, K., Antosiewicz-Bourget, J., Frane, J.L., Tian, S., Nie, J., Jonsdottir, G.A., Ruotti, V., Stewart, R., *et al.* (2007). Induced pluripotent stem cell lines derived from human somatic cells. *Science 318*, 1917-1920.

Yusa, K., Rad, R., Takeda, J., and Bradley, A. (2009). Generation of transgene-free induced pluripotent mouse stem cells by the piggyBac transposon. *Nat Methods 6*, 363-369.

Zhao, H.X., Li, Y., Jin, H.F., Xie, L., Liu, C., Jiang, F., Luo, Y.N., Yin, G.W., Wang, J., Li, L.S., *et al.* (2010). Rapid and efficient reprogramming of human amnion-derived cells into pluripotency by three factors OCT4/SOX2/NANOG. *Differentiation 80*, 123-129.

Zhou, H., Wu, S., Joo, J.Y., Zhu, S., Han, D.W., Lin, T., Trauger, S., Bien, G., Yao, S., Zhu, Y., *et al.* (2009). Generation of induced pluripotent stem cells using recombinant proteins. *Cell Stem Cell 4*, 381-384.

Zhou, Q., Brown, J., Kanarek, A., Rajagopal, J., and Melton, D.A. (2008). In vivo reprogramming of adult pancreatic exocrine cells to beta-cells. *Nature 455*, 627-632.

Zhu, S., Li, W., Zhou, H., Wei, W., Ambasudhan, R., Lin, T., Kim, J., Zhang, K., and Ding, S. (2010). Reprogramming of human primary somatic cells by OCT4 and chemical compounds. *Cell Stem Cell 7*, 651-655.

In: Induced Stem Cells
Editors: P. Sullivan and E. Mortensen
ISBN: 978-1-61324-613-9

Chapter V

Induced Pluripotent Stem Cell Technology for the Study of Neurodegenerative Diseases

***Shiho Kitaoka*[1,2], *Hiroshi Kondoh*[3] *and Haruhisa Inoue*[*1,2,]**
[1]Center for iPS Cell Research and Application (CiRA), Kyoto University, Kyoto, Shogoin, Sakyo-ku, Kyoto, Japan
[2]CREST, JST, Kawaguchi, Saitama, Japan
[3]Department of Geriatric Medicine, Graduate School of Medicine, Kyoto University, Shogoin, Sakyo-ku, Kyoto, Japan

Abstract

Induced pluripotent stem (iPS) cell technology has paved new ways for disease modeling and drug discovery. Disease modeling with the differentiated neuronal cells from patient-specific iPS cells partially recapitulated the phenotypes of spinal muscular atrophy (SMA), familial dysautonomia (FD) and Rett syndrome. Furthermore, proof of the efficacy of candidate drugs by iPS cell-based assay on SMA and FD has been reported.

There are several obstacles for disease modeling using iPS cell-derived neuronal cells. First, differentiated neuronal cells from patient-

* Correspondence (HI): haruhisa@cira.kyoto-u.ac.jp

specific iPS cells might not be provoked sufficiently toward senescence to manifest the phenotype of late-onset diseases such as Parkinson disease (PD) and amyotrophic lateral sclerosis (ALS). Second, there are heterogeneous populations in cultured cells differentiated from iPS cells that might affect the disease phenotype. The propensity of various differentiations among iPS cells leads to the heterogeneity (Figure 1).

In this review, we will describe recent literature concerning the application of iPS cell technology for the study of neurological diseases and also discuss some experimental requirements.

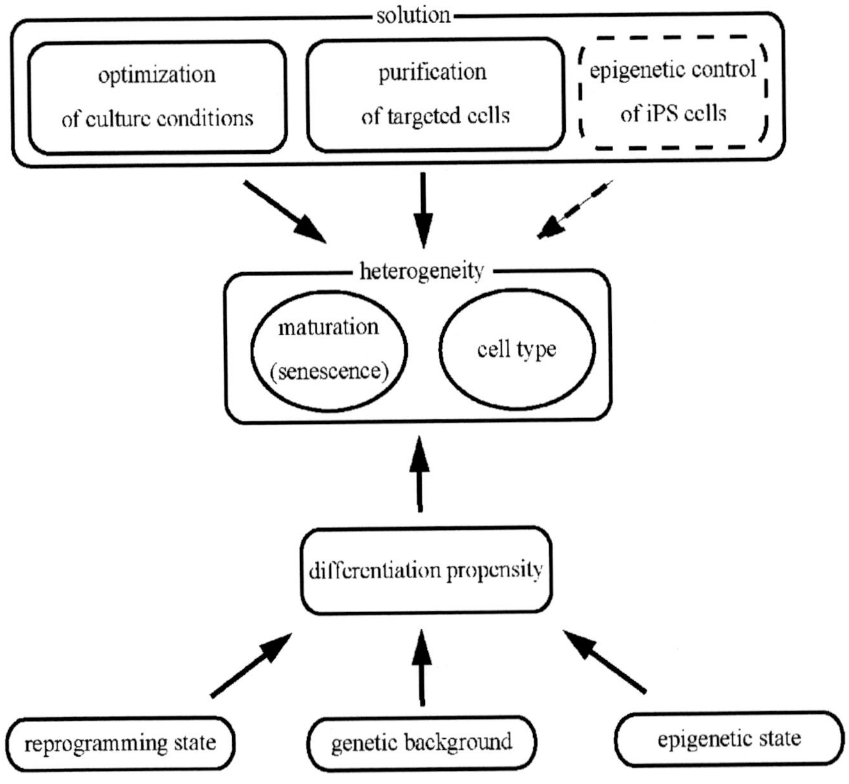

Figure 1. Heterogeneity, including maturation stage and cell population, is a result of the variety of differentiation propensities of iPS cells caused by reprogramming state, genetic background and epigenetic state. Purification of targeted cells and optimization of culture conditions will reduce the heterogeneity and lead to progresses in iPS cell technology.

Introduction

iPS cells are generated by transduction of transcription factors, which are expressed in embryonic stem (ES) cells, in somatic cells (Takahashi *et al.*, 2006; Takahashi *et al.*, 2007; Yu *et al.*, 2007). iPS cells are morphologically identical to ES cells and have the ability to self-renew and differentiate into cells of all germ layers. iPS cell technology makes it possible to analyze *in vitro* affected cell populations that are differentiated from disease-specific iPS cells. This then should enable us to determine the underlying mechanisms of disease, screen new drugs, and develop cell therapy.

Disease phenotypes were partially recapitulated in the differentiated cells from patient-specific iPS cells in some diseases such as spinal muscular atrophy (SMA) (Ebert *et al.*, 2009), familial dysautonomia (FD) (Lee *et al.*, 2009) and Rett syndrome (Marchetto *et al.*, 2010). Furthermore firm evidence of the efficacy of some candidate drugs for SMA (Hastings *et al.*, 2009) and FD (Lee *et al.*, 2009) has also been presented. Other disease phenotypes such as Parkinson's disease (PD) and amyotrophic lateral sclerosis (ALS) have not yet been described in such terms, although midbrain dopaminergic neurons (Soldner *et al.*, 2009) and spinal motor neurons were successfully generated from patient-specific iPS cells (Dimos *et al.*, 2008).

Genetically corrected somatic cells from Fanconi anaemia patients can be reprogrammed to iPS cells (Raya *et al.*, 2009). Further, corrected patient-specific iPS cells can give rise to haematopoietic progenitors of myeloid and erythroid lineages whose phenotypes are normal. This demonstrates the potential value for cell therapy application.

In this review, we will describe recent literature featuring iPS cell technology for the study of neurological diseases, and we will discuss experimental requirements for overcoming several obstacles in disease modeling.

Main Document

iPS Cells Derived from Patients with Neurological Diseases

Since the start of the development of iPS cell technology, disease-specific iPS cell lines were generated from individuals with neurological diseases, as summarized in Table 1. Neurological diseases can be roughly divided into two categories. One includes early-onset, neurodevelopmental diseases such as Rett syndrome (Marchetto *et al.*, 2010), Prader-Willi/Angelman syndrome (Chamberlain *et al.*, 2010), Fragile X syndrome (Urbach *et al.*, 2010), SMA, FD, Friedreich's ataxia (Ku *et al.*, 2010) and Down syndrome (Park *et al.*, 2008). The other includes late-onset, neurodegenerative diseases like ALS, PD and Huntington's disease (Park *et al.*, 2008).

Table 1. Disease-specific iPS cell lines.

	Neurological disease	Primarily affected neuronal population	Control	*in vitro* phenotype	Mutated gene in disease-specific iPS cell
early-onset	Familial dysautonomia (FD)	sensory and autonomic neurons	unaffected	impaired migration	IKBKAP
	Fragile X syndrome	global			FMR1 CGG repeat truncation
	Friedreich's ataxia	sensory neurons	SMA-iPS cells, non-disease unaffected		FXN GAA·TTC repeat expansion
	Angelman syndrome	global	unaffected		15q11-q13 paternal deletion
	Prader-Willi syndrome				15q11-q13 maternal deletion UBE3A
	Down syndrome	global			Trisomy 21
	Rett syndrome	global	unaffected	reduced number of synapses	MeCP2
	Spinal muscular atrophy (SMA)	spinal motor neurons	unaffected mother	motor neuron loss	SMN1
late-onset	Amyotrophic lateral sclerosis (ALS)	motor neurons			SOD1
	Huntington disease (HD)	striatal GABAergic neurons			Huntingtin CAG repeat expansion
	Parkinson disease (PD)	midbrain dopaminergic neurons			

A few of the neurodevelopmental diseases caused by single gene abnormalities resulting in highly penetrant phenotypes were successfully recapitulated with iPS cell technology.

SMA is an autosomal recessive genetic disorder caused by mutations in the survival motor neuron 1 gene (SMN1). Mutations in SMN1 significantly reduce SMN protein expression and result in the selective degeneration of lower motor neurons. Ebert *et al.* (2009) showed that SMA patient-derived spinal motor neurons were reduced in number and cell body size at 6 weeks of differentiation compared to the patient's unaffected mother-derived motor neurons. SMN protein is localized in gems, one of the nuclear compartments, and the number of gems present is inversely correlated to disease severity. The authors detected an increased number of SMN gems in nuclei of both fibroblasts and iPS cells derived from the SMA patient. The homozygous loss of SMN1 is partially compensated for by the presence of another gene, SMN2, which also codes for SMN protein. However, the expression of full-length protein generated from SMN2 is substantially lower than that from SMN1. A single nucleotide replacement of SMN2 compared to SMN1 changes splicing, and that transcript encodes truncated protein. Hastings *et al.* (2009) reported that tetracyclines are able to increase the expression of full-length SMN protein from SMN2 by splicing modulation.

FD is an autosomal recessive genetic disorder caused by mutations in IKBKAP gene involved in transcriptional elongation and characterized by the degeneration of sensory and autonomic neurons. Lee *et al.* (2009) showed marked defects in neurogenic differentiation and impaired migration of neural crest precursor cells derived from FD patients compared to those from non-affected control. Kinetin, one of the plant hormones, increased normal *IKBKAP* and ameliorated neural differentiation and migration.

Rett syndrome is a progressive neurological disorder caused by mutations in X-linked gene encoding MeCP2 protein. Marchetto *et al.* (2010) reported a reduced number of glutamatergic synapses and alteration of morphology in forebrain neurons derived from Rett syndrome patients compared to those from unaffected controls. At 6 weeks of differentiation, neurons from Rett syndrome patients have a significant decrease in frequency and amplitude of spontaneous postsynaptic currents when compared to those from unaffected individuals.

Obstacles of Modeling Late-Onset Neurodegenerative Diseases

A modeling by iPS technology of polygenic, late-onset neurodegenerative diseases has not been reported. Midbrain dopaminergic neurons and spinal cord motor neurons can be differentiated from PD and ALS patient-specific iPS cells, respectively. Perhaps the disease phenotype may never manifest itself under standard culture conditions because differentiated neurons might be too immature or an environment surrounding neurons might differ between *in vitro* (culture) and *in vivo* (brain or spinal cord). It might be revealed by challenging the neural cells with stressors such as oxygen reactive species, proinflammatory factors or co-culture with another type of cell (Marchetto *et al.*, 2008).

Recent investigations have shown that glial cells are affected by physiological brain aging regardless of the absence of any neurodegenerative pathology (Terry *et al.*, 1987). In astrocytes, advanced age initiates conditions similar to mild reactive gliosis. Astroglial cells from advanced-age brain have higher expressions of glial fibrillary acidic protein (GFAP) and glial calcium-bound protein S100 (Le Prince *et al.*, 1993). Additionally, the number of microglial cells is significantly increased (von Bernhardi *et al.*, 2010).

Moreover, the involvement of these non-neuronal cells in neurodegenerative diseases is increasingly being recognized. AD is characterized by profound neuronal loss and prominent reactive astrogliosis and activation of microglia. As Alois Alzheimer suggested, AD plaques are formed by Aβ deposits, degenerating neurites, astroglial processes and activated microglial cells (Vehmas *et al.*, 2002). Activated astrocytes and microglia can release proinflammatory factors such as interleukin-1β and prostaglandin E_2 (Mhatre *et al.*, 2004).

Oxidative stress may play an important role in sporadic PD (Zhang *et al.*, 2000), as it is suggested that patient-derived midbrain dopaminergic neurons might be more vulnerable to oxidative stress.

Identification of new and more effective and relevant stressors or environments that mimic senescence or elicit neuronal phenotypes earlier in models of late-onset neurodegenerative diseases will therefore be a critical goal for future research.

Heterogeneous Population of Differentiated Cells

Although differentiation protocols have been reported for human ES cells and iPS cells in which neural stem cells and specific neuronal or glial cell types are enriched, it has in fact been revealed that heterogeneous cell populations exist under these conditions (Chambers *et al.*, 2009; Hu *et al.*, 2009; Lee *et al.*, 2010). Additionally, cells are not able to synchronize the developmental stage of cell populations to the extent seen in normal development *in vivo*, and consequently cells at different stages of maturation are present in such cultures. Naturally, this cellular heterogeneity impedes experimental and clinical utility.

The purification of specialized cells of interest is essential for recapitulating diseases and transplanting cells. Such procedures will rely on our technique of manipulating iPS cells genetically to express selectable markers under the control of cell type-specific promoters that would utilize fluorescent or magnetic cell sorting (Hockemeyer *et al.*, 2009; Placantonakis *et al.*, 2009).

Genomic insertion of reporter gene has been shown to alter gene function (Kustikova *et al.*, 2005). Therefore, identification of unique combinations of cell surface epitopes can facilitate cell therapy because cells of interest are purified without gene manipulation. Pruszak *et al.* (2007 & 2009) identified the combination of cluster of differentiation (CD) surface antigen code for neural lineage and Elkabetz *et al.* (2008) reported Forse 1 as being a marker for neural rosette cells. However, no markers for region-specific postmitotic neurons have so far been identified.

Inhibition of Notch activity by γ-secretase inhibitor resulted in a marked acceleration of differentiation, thereby shortening the time required for the generation of functionally active human ES cell-derived neurons (Borghese *et al.*, 2010). This kind of inhibitor can eliminate proliferating cells from differentiated neurons to reduce the risk of tumor formation after transplantation.

Resolution of this problem may assist in obtaining more robust phenotypes *in vitro*, finding more effective drugs, and supplying safe cells for cell therapy.

A Variety of Differentiation Propensities of iPS Cells

The generation of iPS cells can be accomplished by employing retroviral vectors to overexpress reprogramming factors. After infected somatic cells are fully reprogrammed into iPS cells, the vectors are silenced. Therefore, the reprogramming state may be evaluated by retroviral vector silencing. However, this viral system has been criticized for its permanent integration of exogenous genes into the genome and their possible involvement in differentiation propensity.

Alternatively, transfection of episomal plasmids or modified RNA was also successful in reprogramming somatic cells (Okita *et al.*, 2010; Yu *et al.*,

2009; Yue *et al.*, 2010; Warren *et al.*, 2010). Moreover, the direct delivery of recombinant protein was also reported to reprogram somatic cells (Zhou *et al.*, 2009). Although these methods eliminate the integrated vector, the gene expression of iPS cells is reflected by that of donor cells (Ghosh *et al.*, 2010). Hence, it is considered that the epigenetic state, including DNA methylation, histone acetylation or histone methylation, may contribute to the differentiation propensities of the respective clones.

Direct conversion from differentiated cells to neurons has been reported (Vierbuchen *et al.*, 2010; Heinrich *et al.*, 2011). This conversion was used to generate mouse subtype-specific neurons from differentiated cells without the need for complete reprogramming to iPS cells. Although this direct conversion is independent from the differentiation propensity of iPS cells, the number of neurons available to study the disease and to be used in high-throughput analysis is limited, and the epigenetic states of these neurons would need to be further analyzed.

Human ES cells are widely variable with regard to epigenetic markers, expression profile and differentiation propensity (Osafune *et al.*, 2008; Rugg-Gunn *et al.*, 2007). And also there is significant intrinsic variance among the iPS cell lines generated to date, as pointed out by Hu *et al.* (2010) & Boulting *et al.* (2011). Pick *et al.* (2009) detected abnormal expression of imprinted genes in a significant number of iPS cell lines. Bock *et al.* (2011) reported that a small set of genes was hypermethylated in iPS cell lines compared to ES cell lines. iPS cells are morphologically similar to ES cells, but the epigenetic state is significantly different between them.

Since there are a variety of methods to generate iPS cells, it is critical for the study of neurodegenerative disease to choose a combination of reprogramming factors, a method of factor delivery, and a cell type to be reprogrammed. For instance, differentiation propensity is partially dependent on the cell type to be reprogrammed (Aoi *et al.*, 2008). For accurate comparison between independent experiments, all conditions should be the same. But there is as yet no standardized parameter for selecting safe and fully reprogrammed iPS cells.

The difficulty of disease modeling is partially attributed to the lack of uniform iPS lines. More robust phenotypes *in vitro* may be obtained in comparison with proper control iPS cell lines.

Conclusion

The development of iPS cell technology has provided both experimental and clinical applications. Once disease-specific phenotypes are identified, this can be translated into cell-based assays for drug screening. However, to accomplish these goals, further improvements are needed. Differentiation methods with higher efficiency will provide larger amounts of cells. The identification of cell surface markers on neuronal or non-neuronal cells will provide homogeneous populations. Highly purified, large amounts of cells of interest will facilitate high-throughput platforms for drug screening. Also crucial is the generation of uniform iPS cells and selection of appropriate iPS cells. This will result in patients having autologous transplantations after their own cells are genetically corrected and/or medicated.

Acknowledgments

We would like to express our sincere gratitude to all our coworkers and collaborators.

Sources of Funding

This study was supported in part by a grant from the Leading Project of MEXT (HI), JST (Japan Science and Technology Agency), CREST (Core Research for Evolutional Science and Technology) (HI), a Grant-in-Aid from the Ministry of Health and Labour (HI), a Grant-in-Aid for Scientific Research (21591079) from JSPS (HI), Grant-in-Aid for Scientific Research (22700377) from JSPS (SK), Grant-in-Aid for Scientific Research on Innovative Area "Foundation of Synapse and Neurocircuit Pathology" (22110007) from the Ministry of Education, Culture, Sports, Science and Technology of Japan (HI), a research grant from the Takeda Science Foundation (HI), a research grant from the Kanae Foundation for the Promotion of Medical Science (HI), and a research grant from the NOVARTIS Foundation for Gerontological Research (HI).

References

Aoi, T., Yae, K., Nakagawa, M., Ichisaka, T., Okita, K., Takahashi, K., Chiba, T. & Yamanaka, S. (2008) Generation of pluripotent stem cells *Science, 321,* 699-702.

Bock, C., Kiskinis, E., Verstappen, G., Gu, H., Boulting, G., Smith, Z. D., Ziller, M., Croft, G. F., Amoroso, M. W., Oakley, D. H., Gnirke, A., Eggan, K. & Meissner, A. (2011) Reference Maps of Human ES and iPS Cell Variation Enable High-Throughput Characterization of Pluripotent Cell Lines. *Cell, 144,* 439-52.

Borghese, L., Dolezalova, D., Opitz, T., Haupt, S., Leinhaas, A., Steinfarz, B., Koch, P., Edenhofer, F., Hampl, A. & Brüstle, O. (2010) Inhibition of notch signaling in human embryonic stem cell-derived neural stem cells delays G1/S phase transition and accelerates neuronal differentiation *in vitro* and *in vivo*. *Stem Cells, 28,* 955-64.

Boulting, G. L., Kiskinis, E., Croft, G. F., Amoroso, M. W., Oakley, D. H., Wainger, B. J., Williams, D. J., Kahler, D. J., Yamaki, M., Davidow, L., Rodolfa, C. T., Dimos, J. T., Mikkilineni, S., Macdermott, A. B., Woolf, C. J., Henderson, C. E., Wichterle, H., Eggan, K. (2011) A functionally characterized test set of human *Nat Biotechnol,* [Epub ahead of print]

Chamberlain SJ, Chen PF, Ng KY, Bourgois-Rocha F, Lemtiri-Chlieh F, Levine ES, Lalande M. (2010) Induced pluripotent stem cell models *Proc Natl Acad Sci U S A., 107,* 17668-73.

Chambers, S. M., Fasano, C. A., Papapetrou, E. P., Tomishima, M., Sadelain, M. & Studer, L. (2009) Highly efficient neural conversion of human ES and iPS cells by dual inhibition of SMAD signaling. *Nat Biotechnol, 27,* 275-80.

Dimos, J. T., Rodolfa, K. T., Niakan, K. K., Weisenthal, L. M., Mitsumoto, H., Chung, W., Croft, G. F., Saphier, G., Leibel, R., Goland, R., Wichterle, H., Henderson, C. E. & Eggan, K. (2008) Induced pluripotent stem cells *Science, 321,* 1218-21.

Ebert, A. D., Yu, J., Rose, F. F., Mattis, V. B., Lorson, C. L., Thomson, J. A. & Svendsen, C. N. (2009) Induced pluripotent stem cells *Nature, 457,* 277-80.

Elkabetz, Y., Panagiotakos, G., Al Shamy, G., Socci, N. D., Tabar, V. & Studer, L. (2008) Human ES cell-derived neural rosettes reveal a functionally distinct early neural stem cell stage. *Genes Dev, 22,* 152-65.

Ghosh, Z., Wilson, K. D., Wu, Y., Hu, S., Quertermous, T. & Wu, J. C. (2010) Persistent donor cell gene expression among human induced pluripotent stem cells contributes to differences with human embryonic stem cells. *PLoS One, 5,* e8975.

Hastings, M. L., Berniac, J., Liu, Y. H., Abato, P., Jodelka, F. M., Barthel, L., Kumar, S., Dudley, C., Nelson, M., Larson., Edmonds, J., Bowser, T., Draper, M., Higgins, P. & Krainer, A. R. (2009) Tetracyclines that promote SMN2 exon 7 splicing as therapeutics for spinal muscular atrophy. *Sci Transl Med, 1,* 1-10.

Heinrich, C., Gascón, S., Masserdotti, G., Lepier, A., Sanchez, R., Simon-Ebert, T., Schroeder, T., Götz, M. & Berninger, B. (2011) Generation of subtype-specific neurons from postnatal astroglia of the mouse cerebral cortex. *Nat Protoc, 6,* 214-28.

Hockemeyer, D., Soldner, F., Beard, C., Gao, Q., Mitalipova, M., DeKelver, R. C., Katibah, G. E., Amora, R., Boydston, E. A., Zeitler, B., Meng, X., Miller, J. C., Zhang, L., Rebar, E. J., Gregory, P. D., Urnov, F. D. & Jaenisch, R. (2009) Efficient targeting of expressed and silent genes *Nat Biotechnol, 27,* 851-7.

Hu, B. Y., Du, Z.W. & Zhang, S.C. (2009) Differentiation of human oligodendrocytes from pluripotent stem cells. *Nat Protoc, 4,* 1614-22.

Hu, B. Y., Weick, J. P., Yu, J., Ma, L. X., Zhang, X. Q., Thomson, J. A. & Zhang, S. C. (2010) Neural differentiation of human induced pluripotent stem cells follows developmental principles but with variable potency. *Proc Natl Acad Sci U S A, 107,* 4335-40.

Ku, S., Soragni, E., Campau, E., Thomas, E. A., Altun, G., Laurent, L. C., Loring, J. F., Napierala, M. & Gottesfeld, J. M. (2010) Friedreich's ataxia *Cell Stem Cell, 7,* 631-7.

Kustikova, O., Fehse, B., Modlich, U., Yang, M., Düllmann, J., Kamino., von Neuhoff, N., Schlegelberger, B., Li, Z. & Baum, C. (2005) Clonal dominance of hematopoietic stem cells triggered by retroviral gene marking. *Science, 308,* 1171-4.

Le Prince, G., Delaere, P., Fages, C., Duyckaerts, C., Hauw, J. J. & Tardy, M. (1993) Alterations of glial fibrillary acidic *Neurosci Lett, 151,* 71-3.

Lee, G., Papapetrou, E. P., Kim, H., Chambers, S. M., Tomishima, M. J., Fasano, C. A., Ganat, Y. M., Menon, J., Shimizu, F., Viale, A., Tabar, V., Sadelain, M. & Studer, L. (2009) Modelling pathogenesis and treatment of familial dysautonomia using patient-specific iPSCs. *Nature, 461,* 402-6.

Lee, G., Chambers, S. M., Tomishima, M. J. & Studer, L. (2010) Derivation of neural crest cells from human pluripotent stem cells. *Nat Protoc, 5,* 688-701.

Marchetto, M. C., Muotri, A. R., Mu, Y., Smith, A. M., Cezar, G. G. & Gage. (2008) Non-cell-autonomous effect of human SOD1 G37R astrocytes on motor neurons derived from human embryonic stem cells. *Cell Stem Cell, 3,* 649-57.

Marchetto, M. C., Carromeu, C., Acab, A., Yu, D., Yeo, G. W., Mu, Y., Chen, G., Gage, F. H. & Muotri, A. R. (2010) A model for neural development *Cell, 143,* 527-39.

Mhatre, M., Floyd, R. A. & Hensley, K. (2004) Oxidative stress *J Alzheimers Dis, 6,* 147-57.

Okita, K., Hong, H., Takahashi, K. & Yamanaka, S. (2010) Generation of mouse-induced pluripotent stem cells Nat Protoc, 5, 418-28.

Osafune, K., Caron, L., Borowiak, M., Martinez, R. J., Fitz-Gerald, C. S., Sato, Y., Cowan, C. A., Chien, K. R. & Melton, D. A. (2008) Marked differences in differentiation propensity among human *Nat Biotechnol, 26,* 313-5.

Park, I. H., Arora, N., Huo, H., Maherali, N., Ahfeldt, T., Shimamura, A., Lensch, M. W., Cowan, C., Hochedlinger, K. & Daley, G. Q. (2008) Disease-specific induced pluripotent stem cells. *Cell, 134,* 877-86.

Pick, M., Stelzer, Y., Bar-Nur, O., Mayshar, Y., Eden, A. & Benvenisty, N. (2009) Clone- and gene-specific aberrations of parental imprinting in human induced pluripotent stem cells. *Stem Cells, 27,* 2686-90.

Placantonakis, D. G., Tomishima, M. J., Lafaille, F., Desbordes, S. C., Jia, F., Socci, N. D., Viale, A., Lee, H., Harrison, N., Tabar, V. & Studer, L. (2009) BAC transgenesis in human embryonic stem cells as a novel tool to define the human neural lineage. *Stem Cells, 27,* 521-32.

Pruszak, J., Sonntag, K. C., Aung, M. H., Sanchez-Pernaute, R. & Isacson, O. (2007) Markers and methods for cell sorting of human *Stem Cells, 25,* 2257-68.

Pruszak, J., Ludwig, W., Blak, A., Alavian, K. & Isacson, O. (2009) CD15, CD24, and CD29 define a surface biomarker code for neural lineage differentiation of stem cells *Stem Cells, 27,* 2928-40.

Raya, A., Rodríguez-Pizà, I., Guenechea, G., Vassena, R., Navarro, S., Barrero, M. J., Consiglio, A., Castellà, M., Río, P., Sleep, E., González, F., Tiscornia, G., Garreta, E., Aasen, T., Veiga, A., Verma, I. M., Surrallés, J., Bueren, J. & Izpisúa Belmonte, J. C. (2009) Disease-corrected haematopoietic progenitors from Fanconi anaemia induced pluripotent stem cells *Nature, 460,* 53-59.

Rugg-Gunn, P. J., Ferguson-Smith, A. C. & Pedersen, R. A. (2007) Status of genomic imprinting in human embryonic stem cells as revealed by a large cohort of independently derived and maintained lines. *Hum Mol Genet, 16,* R243-51.

Soldner, F., Hockemeyer, D., Beard, C., Gao, Q., Bell, G. W., Cook, E. G., Hargus, G., Blak, A., Cooper, O., Mitalipova, M., Isacson, O. & Jaenisch, R. (2009) Parkinson's disease patient-derived induced pluripotent stem cells free of viral reprogramming factors. *Cell, 136,* 964-77.

Takahashi, K. & Yamanaka, S. (2006) Induction of pluripotent stem cells from mouse embryonic and adult fibroblast cultures by defined factors. *Cell, 126,* 663-76.

Takahashi, K., Tanabe, K., Ohnuki, M., Narita, M., Ichisaka, T., Tomoda, K. & Yamanaka, S. (2007) Induction of pluripotent stem cells *Cell, 131,* 861-72.

Terry, R. D., DeTeresa, R. & Hansen, L. A. (1987) Neocortical cell counts in normal human adult aging. *Ann Neurol, 21,* 530-9.

Urbach, A., Bar-Nur, O., Daley, G. Q. & Benvenisty, N. (2010) Differential modeling of fragile X syndrome by human embryonic stem cells and induced pluripotent stem cells. *Cell Stem Cell, 6,* 407-11.

Vehmas AK, Kawas CH, Stewart WF, Troncoso JC. (2003) Immune reactive cells in senile plaques and cognitive decline in Alzheimer's disease. *Neurobiol Aging, 24,* 321-31.

Vierbuchen, T., Ostermeier, A., Pang, Z. P., Kokubu, Y., Südhof, T. C. & Wernig, M. (2010) Direct conversion of fibroblasts to functional neurons by defined factors. *Nature, 463,* 1035-41.

von Bernhardi, R., Tichauer, J. E. & Eugenín, J. (2010) Aging-dependent changes of microglial cells and their relevance *J Neurochem, 112,* 1099-114.

Warren, L., Manos, P. D., Ahfeldt, T., Loh, Y. H., Li, H., Lau, F., Ebina, W., Mandal, P. K., Smith, Z. D., Meissner, A., Daley, G. Q., Brack, A. S., Collins, J. J., Cowan, C., Schlaeger, T. M. & Rossi, D. J. (2010) Highly efficient reprogramming to pluripotency and directed differentiation of human *Cell Stem Cell, 7,* 618-30.

Yu, J., Vodyanik, M. A., Smuga-Otto, K., Antosiewicz-Bourget, J., Frane, J. L., Tian, S., Nie, J., Jonsdottir, G. A., Ruotti, V., Stewart, R., Slukvin, I. I. & Thomson, J. A. (2007) Induced pluripotent stem cell lines derived from human somatic cells. *Science, 318,* 1917-20.

Yu, J., Hu, K., Smuga-Otto, K., Tian, S., Stewart, R., Slukvin, II. & Thomson, J. A. (2009) Human induced pluripotent stem cells *Science, 324,* 797-801.

Yue XS, Fujishiro M, Toyoda M, Akaike T, Ito Y. (2010) Reprogramming of somatic cells induced by fusion of embryonic stem cells using hemagglutinating virus of Japan envelope (HVJ-E). *Biochem Biophys Res Commun*, 394, 1053-7.

Zhang, Y., Dawson, V. L. & Dawson, T. M. (2000) Oxidative stress *Neurobiol Dis, 7,* 240-50.

In: Induced Stem Cells
Editors: P. Sullivan and E. Mortensen

ISBN: 978-1-61324-613-9

Chapter VI

Generation of Human Induced Pluripotent Stem Cells from Cord Blood Cells

Naoki Nishishita[1,2], *Chiemi Takenaka*[1,2], *Noemi Fusaki*[3] *and Shin Kawamata*[*1,2]
[1]Foundation for Biomedical Research and Innovation, Chuo-ku, Japan
[2]RIKEN, Center for Developmental Biology, Chuo-ku, Japan
[3]DNAVEC. corp., JST PRESTO, Tsukuba City, Ibaraki Japan

Abstract

We report that iPS cells can be safely and effectively generated from fresh human cord blood (CB) cells with Sendai virus (SeV) vector carrying reprogramming factors *OCT3/4, SOX2, KLF4,* and *c-MYC*. The SeV vector is a single strand RNA virus having no DNA phase, and selectively infects the freshly isolated $CD34^+$ $CD45^{low+}$ fraction of CB cells corresponding to hematopoietic progenitors. Approximately twenty ES cell-like colonies emerged from 1 X 10^4 freshly isolated $CD34^+$ CB cells around 18 days after SeV infection and were selected for passage to reduce the frequency of the remaining SeV-infected cells. The complete elimination of viral constructs was confirmed after several passages by

* corresponding author: kawamata@fbri.org

immunostaining with monoclonal antibody against hemagglutinin-neuraminidase (HN) and by RT-PCR analysis. Five ES cell-like clones were selected to examine their *in vitro* potential for three germ layer differentiation and their capacity for teratoma formation. Generation of non-integrating Sendai virus (SeV) iPS cells from CB cells may be an important step to provide allogeneic iPS cell-derived therapy in the future.

Keywords : CD34+ cells, cord blood, induced pluripotent stem cells (iPSc), Sendai virus (SeV)

Introduction

Since the first report of mouse induced pluripotent stem (iPS) cells by retroviral vectors (1) in 2006, other exogenous gene delivery systems such as adenoviruses (2), sendai viruses (3), conventional plasmids (4), the piggyBac transposition system (5, 6), Cre-excisable viruses (7) and the oriP/EBNA1-episomal vector (8) have been reported. Further, protein delivery methods (9, 10) and small molecule delivery methods (11, 12) have been reported to explore "safer" iPS cell generation methods. Importantly, the efficiency of generating iPS cells differs greatly depending on the reagents, methods, and cell sources used.

As for the cell source for generating iPS cells, a variety of cell types or tissues have been reported, including dermal fibroblasts (1), keratinocytes (13), hepatocytes (14), $CD34^+$ peripheral blood cells (15), thymocytes (16) and $CD34^+$ cord blood (CB) cells (17,18). However, among these, CB cells have advantages over other cell sources. Unlike the cells or tissues obtained by sampling or biopsy from a variety of organs at different ages, freshly isolated (non-cultured) $CD34^+$ CB cells have distinct genetic and epigenetic profiles as hematopoietic stem cells and progenitors. Further, this fraction is the youngest stem cell population available following birth and is free from post-natal individual genomic or epigenetic alterations caused by chemicals and / or UV irradiation and also free from genetic deletions related to rearrangements of the T/B cell receptor. Thus, generating iPS cells from this fraction facilitates our understanding of the reprogramming process by knowing the genetic profile of the cell source ($CD34^+$ CB cells), and the reprogrammed cells (iPS cells). Further, it is possible to collaborate with existing public cord banks that preserve CB cells in a clinical setting with individual HLA-typing information.

There are technical advantages in the use of SeV vectors for the efficient reprogramming of cells. Being a single strand RNA virus, Sendai virus makes use of sialic acid residues on surface glycoproteins or asialoglycoproteins present on most cell types for cell entry and will not integrate into DNA of the host cells throughout replication processes.

In this chapter, we show the methods for reprogramming $CD34^+$ CB cells with Sendai virus vector and the maintenance of the established iPS cells with or without feeder cells.

1. Reprogramming of $CD34^+$ Cells from Cord Blood.

Fresh CB cells for research use were procured from Asagiri Hospital after obtaining approval of the ethics committee of Asagiri Hospital. Frozen $CD34^+$ CB cells were supplied by Riken BioResource Center (Riken BRC, Tsukuba Japan). All the experiments, including animal studies, were reviewed and approved by the ethics committees of institutions with which the authors were affiliated.

Section 1.1. Purification of Mononuclear Cells from CB Cells

Mononuclear cells were isolated from fresh CB cells with Lymphoprep TM (Cosmo Bio Co. Tokyo, Japan) in accordance with the manufacturer's instructions. Around 0.3 - 0.8% of mononuclear cells expressed CD34 and this fraction also expressed CD45 antigen at low levels and corresponded to a population containing hematopoietic stem cells and progenitors. Interestingly, Sendai virus (SeV) selectively infected this freshly isolated fraction (Figure 1 A, C). Based on this finding, purified $CD34^+$ cells were used as a cell source for reprogramming with Sendai virus (Figure 1 B).

Section 1.2. Introduction of Reprogramming Factors to $CD34^+$ CB Cells with Sev

The $CD34^+$ cells were cultured for one day in hematopoietic culture (HC) media [serum-free X-VIVO10 (Lonza, Basel Switzerland) containing 50 ng/mL IL-6 (Peprotech, London UK), 50 ng/mL sIL-6R (Peprotech), 50 ng/mL SCF (Peprotech), 10 ng/mL TPO (Peprotech), 20 ng/mL Flt3-ligand (R&D system, MN)] in six well plates at a density of 2 X 10^4 cells / 2 mL / well before the infection with SeV. Sendai virus vector constructs inserting four reprogramming factors and GFP (SeV18+ HS-*OCT3/4*/TS⊿F, SeV18+HS-*SOX2*/TS⊿F, SeV18+ HS-*KLF4*/TS⊿F, SeV *(HNL)c-MYC*/TS15⊿F, SeV18+*GFP*/TS⊿F) were supplied by DNAVEC Corp. The $CD34^+$ cells (1 x 10^4) were transferred to 96 well plates in 180 μL of hematopoietic cell culture media with 20 μL of viral supernatant containing 1-10 m.o.i. of SeV constructs (Figure 2). The HC medium was changed with fresh media the following day and infected cells were cultured for another four days.

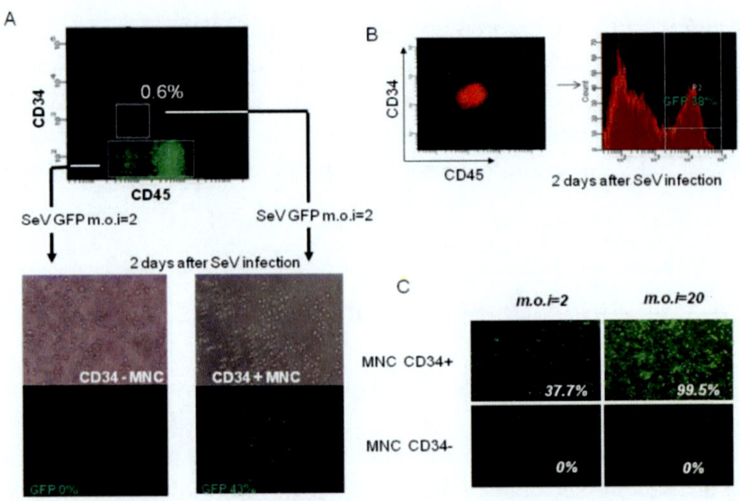

Figure 1. SeV selectively infects $CD34^+$ CB cells. A: Freshly isolated mononuclear cells were infected with Sendai virus (SeV, 2 m.o.i) and fractionated by CD34 expression with a cell sorter (upper panel). The microscopic and fluorescence observations of $CD34^{+/-}$ sorted fractions two days after infection are shown in the lower panels. The percentage of GFP expression determined by flow cytometry is appended in photos. B: Flow cytometric analysis of CD34 and CD45 expression of $CD34^+$ purified cells (Riken BRC) to be reprogrammed is shown in dot pot (left panel). Infection efficiency of 2 m.o.i. SeV with $CD34^+$ cells two days after infection was evaluated by flow cytometry (histogram, right panel). C: Infection efficiency of SeV in $CD34^+$ cells increases up to 99% if higher titers (20 m.o.i.) of Sev are applied. The percentages of GFP expression with 2 or 20 m.o.i. SeV determined by flow cytometry are appended in photos.

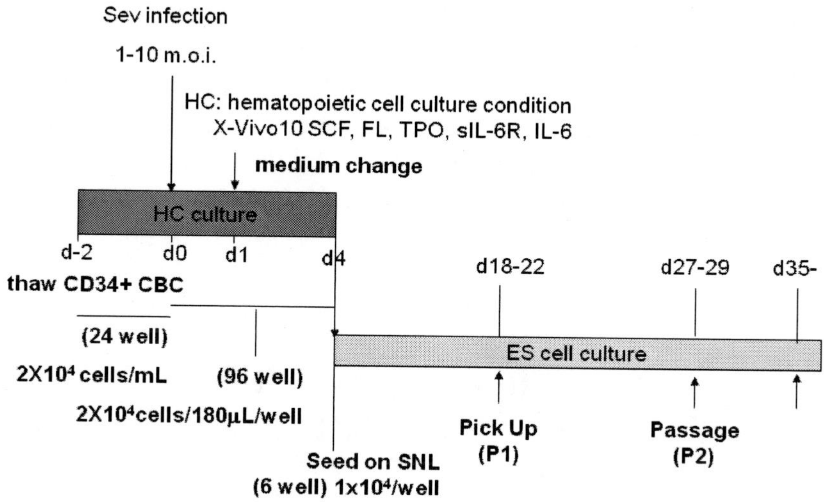

Figure 2. Schema for generation of virus-free iPS cells from $CD34^+$ CB cells with SeV vector. ES cell-like colonies were picked up around three weeks after seeding on SNL. Cell clumps from colonies were seeded on SNL to determine the ability for serial passages and further appraisal of reprogrammed cells.

Section 1.3. Generation of ES-Like Cells on Feeder Cells

Preparation of feeder (MMC-SNL) cells: SNL76/7 cells (European Collection of Cell Culture, Salisbury, UK) were cultured in 10% FBS/DMEM and treated with 100 μL of mitomycin C solution (1 mg/mL) (Nacalai Tesque, Kyoto, Japan) in 10 cm dishes for three hours to generate mitomycin C treated-SNL 76/7 feeder cells (MMC-SNL).

*Preparation of human ES cell media:*_DMEM/F-12-based medium (SIGMA) containing 20% KSR (Invitrogen), 2 mM L-glutamine (Invitrogen), 1% NEAA (Invitrogen), 0.1 mM 2-ME (Invitrogen), 4 ng/mL bFGF (Peprotech) was freshly prepared every time before use.

Ten thousand CB cells were seeded on MMC-SNL in six well plates in human ES cell media under 20% O_2 culture conditions. The human ES cell medium was changed every 48-60 hours. ES cell-like colonies emerged 18 - 22 days after initiating co-culture on MMC-SNL. Emergent colonies were mechanically picked up with a Pipetman and transferred onto a 24 well plate preseeded with MMC-SNL to test for serial passage. Usually, ten colonies were picked from a 24 well plate for further appraisal for pluripotency (Figure

2). For colony passage, a 96 well plate with 180 μL ES cell medium without feeder cells was used to monitor both cell clump size (small cell clumps with a 30 – 50 μm diameter) and number. One cell clump was transferred to one well for passage. The cells were incubated until the colony size reached 500 μm in diameter (P1). The medium was changed every day. After culturing the cell colony on the 24 well plate for five to seven days, the emergent colonies were transferred to a six well plate pre-seeded with MMC-SNL (P2). The split ratio was routinely 1:3 or 1:4.

2. Establishment of iPS Cells from $CD34^+$ CB Cells

Section 2.1. Immunohistological Staining of ES Cell-Like Clones

ES cell like-colonies were tested for alkaline phosphatase activities with the Leukocyte Alkaline Phosphatase kit (VECTOR, Burlingame, CA) in accordance with the manufacturer's instructions. For immunochemical staining, colonies were fixed with 4% paraformaldehyde followed by staining with a series of antibodies listed in Table 1. Nuclei were stained with DAPI (1:1000, SIGMA). Photomicrographs were taken with a fluorescent microscope (Olympus BX51, IX71, Tokyo) and a visible light microscope (Olympus CKX31) (Figure 3, panels A - I).

Table 1. Antibodies for Immunochemical staining.

Antibodies	supplier	Cat No	Dilution
anti-Oct4	Santa Cruz	sc-5279	1/100
anti-TRA-1-81	Chemicon	MAB4381	1/200
anti-TRA-1-60	Chemicon	MAB4360	1/200
anti-SSEA-3	Chemicon	MAB4303	1/200
anti-SSEA-4	Chemicon	MAB4304	1/200
anti-Nanog	Reprocell	RCAB0003P	1/1000
a-fetoprotein(AFP)	R&D	MAB1368	1/100
desmin	Dako	M0760	1/50
beta-III tubulin	SIGMA	T4026	1/200

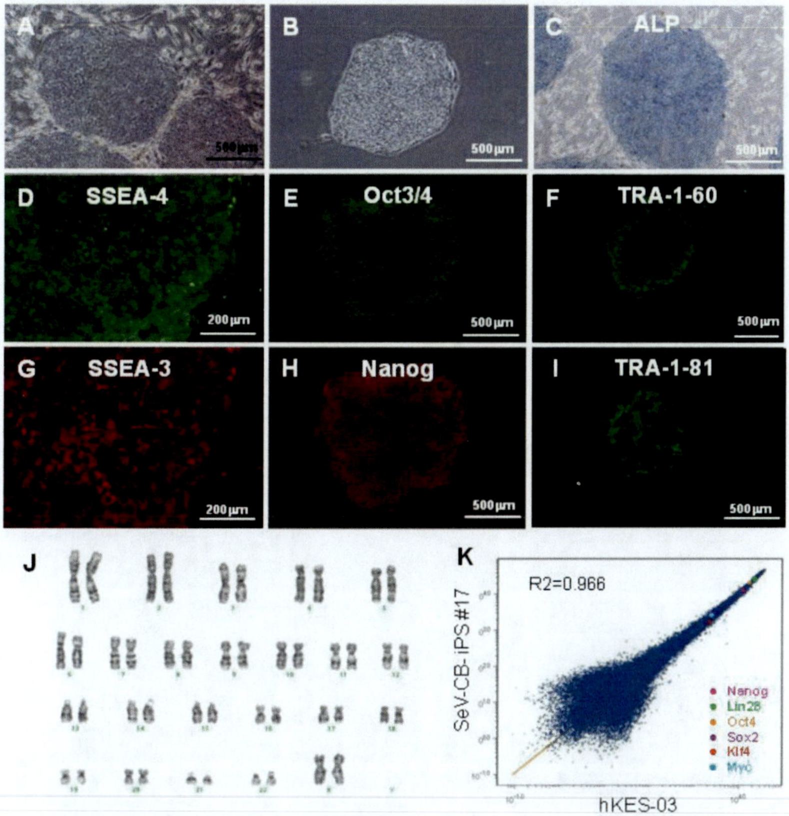

Figure 3. Expression of pluripotency-associated molecules in reprogrammed cells. Phase contrast images of a representative virus free ES cell like colony on SNL (A), on Matrigel (B). Established cell line SeV-CB-iPS clone #17 was stained for ALP activities (C), SSEA-4 (D), Oct3/4 (E), TRA-1-60 (F), SSEA-3 (G), Nanog (H) and TRA-1-81 (I). Alexa 594 (red) and Alexa 488 (green) conjugated secondary antibodies were used to visualize expression (D-I). Karyotype analysis of SeV-CB-iPS clone #17 (J) and gene expression profile of SeV-CB-iPS clone #17 compared with human ES cell line KhES-3 is shown in panel K.

Section 2.2. Karyotype and Gene Chip Analysis of an ES Cell-Like Clone

The karyotype of ES cell-like clones was reported by an out-sourcing laboratory (Nihon Gene Research Laboratories Inc., Sendai, Japan). The karyotypes of 50 cells were analyzed by G-band staining. After 15 passages,

ES cell-like clone SeV-CB-iPS#17 exhibited a normal karyotype (46 XY, Figure 3 J). Total RNA from several reprogrammed cell clones, the human ES cell line KhES-3 (a gift from Yamanaka's lab, Kyoto University), $CD34^+$ CB cells and CB mononuclear cells were extracted with RNeasy Mini kit (QIAGEN) and hybridized with human Gene Chip (U133 plus 2.0 Array Affymetrix) according to the manufacturer's instructions (Figure 3K).

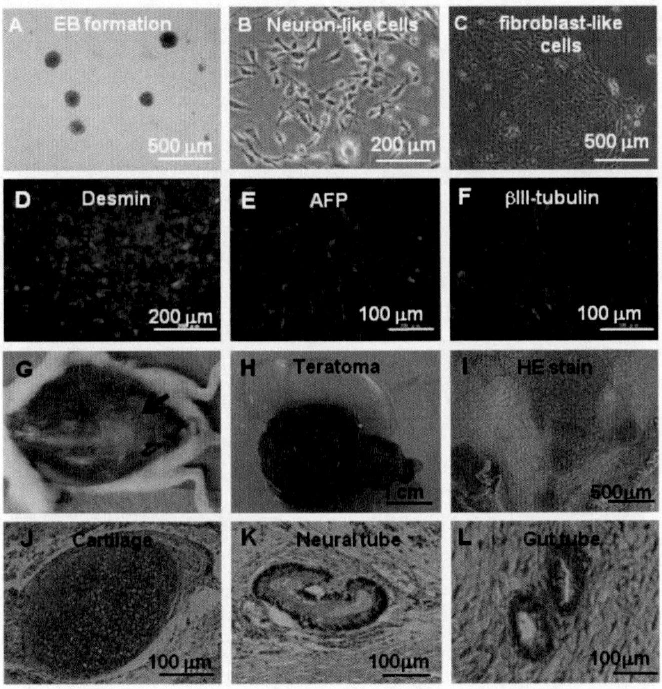

Figure 4. *In vitro* and *in vivo* differentiation potentials of reprogrammed cell line. Embryoid body-mediated differentiation of reprogrammed cells line SeV-CB-iPS clone #17 (A-F). Bright field images of embryoid body generated after eight days of culture (A). Embryoid bodies were transferred to gelatin dishes and differentiated for a further eight days to induce either undirected or guided differentiation (B-F). Phase contrast images of neuron-like cells (B) and fibroblast-like cells (C) after differentiation on gelatin. Cells were fixed and stained for desmin (D:mesoderm differentiation), AFP (E:endoderm differentiation) and βIII-tubulin (F:ectoderm differentiation) to determine lineage-specific differentiation potential. Teratoma formed from SeV-CB-iPS clone #17 (G-L). SCID mice with teratoma (G). Appearance of teratoma (H), Hematoxylin and eosin staining of teratoma derived from iPS cells at low magnification (I). Histology showed derivatives of all three embryonic germ layers including a cartilage-like (J: mesoderm), neural rosette-like (K: ectoderm) and gut-like epithelium (L: endoderm) tissue.

Section 2.3 Differentiation Potential of ES Cell-Like Clones *In Vitro* and *In Vivo*

The three germ layer differentiation potential of the reprogrammed CB cells *in vitro* was determined by placing cells in various culture differentiation conditions. In addition, the three germ layer differentiation potential was determined *in vivo* by injecting one million reprogrammed cells beneath the testicular capsule of SCID mice to form teratomas consisting of all three germ layers. The cell's ability for differentiation to all three germ layers is essential to define a reprogrammed cell as an "induced pluripotent stem" (iPS) cell.

Protocol for Differentiation Potential of Reprogrammed Cells In Vitro

In Vitro Differentiation of reprogrammed cells on gelatin-coated plates: Reprogrammed CB cells were harvested using collagenase IV. Cell clumps (30 – 50 μm) were transferred to six well ultra low attachment plates (Corning) and cultured in DMEM/F12 containing 20% knockout serum replacement (KSR, Invitrogen), 2 mM L-glutamine, 1% NEAA (Invitrogen), 0.1 mM 2-ME (Invitrogen), and 0.5% penicillin and streptomycin (Invitrogen) to form embryoid bodies (EB). The medium was changed every other day. The resulting EBs were transferred to gelatin-coated plates after eight days and cultured in the same fresh medium for another eight days.

Protocol for Differentiation Potential of Reprogrammed Cells In Vivo

Over one million iPS cells were injected beneath the testicular capsule of SCID mice (SLC Japan) for teratoma formation. Tumor formation was observed 60 - 80 days after cell transplantation. Tumor tissues were fixed with 3% formalin followed by staining with hematoxylin and eosin.

3. Maintenance of CB Cell-Derived iPS Cells

Section 3.1. Maintenance of ips Cells On Feeder Cells

iPS cell colonies were cultured in a six well plate preseeded with MMC-SNL until colonies reached 70 - 80% confluency. For passage of colonies,

SNL feeder cells were removed by incubating the colonies with CTK solution at 37°C for three to five min. Then, detached iPS cell clumps were pipetted to reduce the size to 30 – 50 μm diameter and suspended in fresh human ES cell medium to transfer either to a 100 mm dish or six well plate pre-seeded with MMC-SNL cells. The medium was changed every day.

Section 3.2. Maintenance of ips Cells without Feeder Cells

Preparation of MatrigelTM-coated culture dishes: Matrigel™-coated culture dishes were made by first dissolving 1.0 mL of Matrigel™ (BD Bioscience) in 50 mL of distilled DMEM-F12 medium. The culture plate was coated by adding enough Matrigel™ solution to cover the entire bottom of the dish. For example, five mL of Matrigel™ solution was used for a 100 mm dish or a six well plate. The dish or plate was incubated with Matrigel™ for at least 15 min at room temperature, after which excess Matrigel™ solution was aspirated. To start the culture, iPS cell clumps were seeded on the Matrigel™ -coated 100 mm dish or six well plate and incubated until colonies reached 70 - 80% confluency. The 50 -100 μm iPS cell clumps were harvested using CTK solutions and approximately 1.0 x 10^6 cells were transferred to Matrigel™ coated-100 mm dishes or six well plates.

Acknowledgments

We thank M. Shikamura, N. Takada, and K. Matsushima for animal study and maintenance of iPS clones. We also thank S.I. Nishikawa, S. Nishikawa, and K. Kobayashi for useful discussions and supervision of animal experiments and M. Miyako for typing and editorial help. We also thank T. Aoi for supplying total RNA from the hES cell line KhES-3 and Riken BCR for supplying $CD34^+$ CB cells. This work was partly supported by a grant from the Grant-in-Aid for JSPS Fellows 2210853 and S-Innovation project JST Tokyo Japan (2009-2011).

References

[1] Takahashi, K., Yamanaka, S. Induction of pluripotent stem cells *Cell*, 2006, 126: 663-76.

[2] Stadtfeld M, Nagaya M, Utikal J, Weir G, Hochedlinger K. Induced 2 pluripotent stem cells generated without viral integration. *Science*, 2008, 322: 945–949.

[3] Fusaki, N., Ban, H., Nishiyama, A., Saeki, K., and Hasegawa, M. Efficient induction of transgene-free human pluripotent stem cells using a vector based on Sendai virus, an RNA virus that does not integrate into the host genome. *Proc Jpn Acad Ser B Phys Biol Sci*. 2009, 85, 348-362.

[4] Okita, K., Nakagawa, M., Hyenjong, H., Ichisaka, T., and Yamanaka, S. Generation of mouse induced pluripotent stem cells without viral vectors. *Science*, 2008, 322, 949-953.

[5] Woltjen, K., Michael, I. P., Mohseni, P., Desai, R., Mileikovsky, M., Hamalainen, R., Cowling, R., Wang, W., Liu, P., Gertsenstein, M., et al. piggyBac transposition reprograms fibroblasts to induced pluripotent stem cells. *Nature*, 2009, 458, 766-770.

[6] Kaji, K., Norrby, K., Paca, A., Mileikovsky, M., Mohseni, P., and Woltjen, K. Virus-free induction of pluripotency and subsequent excision of reprogramming factors. *Nature*, 2009, 458, 771-775.

[7] Soldner, F., Hockemeyer, D., Beard, C., Gao, Q., Bell, G. W., Cook, E. G., Hargus, G., Blak, A., Cooper, O., Mitalipova, M., et al. Parkinson's disease patient-derived induced pluripotent stem cells free of viral reprogramming factors. *Cell*, 2009, 136, 964-977.

[8] Yu, J., Hu, K., Smuga-Otto, K., Tian, S., Stewart, R., Slukvin, II, and Thomson, J. A.. Human induced pluripotent stem cells free of vector and transgene sequences. *Science*, 2009, 324, 797-801.

[9] Zhou, H., Wu, S., Joo, J. Y., Zhu, S., Han, D. W., Lin, T., Trauger, S., Bien, G., Yao, S., Zhu, Y., et al. Generation of induced pluripotent stem cells using recombinant proteins. *Cell Stem Cell*, 2009, 4, 381-384.

[10] Kim, D., Kim, C. H., Moon, J. I., Chung, Y. G., Chang, M. Y., Han, B. S., Ko, S., Yang, E., Cha, K. Y., Lanza, R., and Kim, K. S. Generation of human induced pluripotent stem cells by direct delivery of reprogramming proteins. *Cell Stem Cell*, 2009, 4, 472-476.

[11] Li, W., Wei, W., Zhu, S., Zhu, J., Shi, Y., Lin, T., Hao, E., Hayek, A., Deng, H., and Ding, S.. Generation of rat and human induced pluripotent stem cells by combining genetic reprogramming and chemical inhibitors. *Cell Stem Cell,* 2009, 4, 16-19.

[12] Huangfu, D., Maehr, R., Guo, W., Eijkelenboom, A., Snitow, M., Chen, A. E., and Melton, D. A.. Induction of pluripotent stem cells by defined factors is greatly improved by small-molecule compounds. *Nat Biotechnol*, 2008, 26, 795-797.

[13] Aasen, T., Raya, A., Barrero, M. J., Garreta, E., Consiglio, A., Gonzalez, F., Vassena, R., Bilic, J., Pekarik, V., Tiscornia, G., et al. Efficient and rapid generation of induced pluripotent stem cells from human keratinocytes. *Nat Biotechnol*, 2008, 26, 1276-1284.

[14] Liu H, Ye Z, Kim Y, Sharkis S, Jang YY., Generation of endoderm *Hepatology*, 2010, 51,1810-9.

[15] Loh, Y. H., Agarwal, S., Park, I. H., Urbach, A., Huo, H., Heffner, G. C., Kim, K., Miller, J. D., Ng, K., and Daley, G. Q. Generation of induced pluripotent stem cells from human blood. *Blood*, 2009,113, 5476-5479.

[16] Hashimoto, H., Kodaira, M., et al. Generation of induced pluripotent stem cells from human terminally differentiated circulating T cells. *Cell Stem Cell*, 2010, 7, 11-14.

[17] Takenaka, C., Nishishita, N., Takada, N., Jakt, L. M., and Kawamata, S.. Effective generation of iPS cells from CD34+ cord blood cells by inhibition of p53. *Exp Hematol,* 2010, 38, 154-162.

[18] Giorgetti, A., Montserrat, N., Aasen, T., Gonzalez, F., Rodriguez-Piza, I., Vassena, R., Raya, A., Boue, S., Barrero, M. J., Corbella, B. A., et al. Generation of induced pluripotent stem cells from human cord blood using OCT4 and SOX2. *Cell Stem Cell,* 2009, 5, 353-357.

Index

A

B

C

D

E

F

G

H

I

J

K

L

M

N

O

P

Q

R

S

T

U

V

W

Y